PREPAREDNESS
Now! ☑

PREPAREDNESS *now!* ☑

[AN EMERGENCY SURVIVAL GUIDE]
REVISED EDITION

ATON EDWARDS

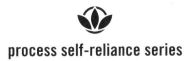

process self-reliance series

PREPAREDNESS NOW! is part of the Process Self-Reliance Series

Process Media
1240 W. Sims Way Suite 124
Port Townsend, WA 98368
www.processmediainc.com

Cover design by Lissi Irwin
Interior Design by Bill Smith
Illustrations by Gregg Einhorn
ISBN 978-1-934170-09-0
Printed in the United States of America
10 9 8 7 6 5 4

PREPAREDNESS NOW!

is dedicated to my wonderful son, Amen.
Daddy loves you.

Table of Contents

Table of Contents continued

From the Publishers

HURRICANE KATRINA AND 9/11 WERE WAKE-UP CALLS; AUTHORITIES TELL US THAT when disaster strikes, everyone must be able to fend for themselves for at least three days. This book is for those who may have once believed preparedness to be unnecessary but now understand it is an essential foundation for informed and responsible living in the 21st Century.

Author Aton Edwards, Founder of International Preparedness Network, has trained thousands in emergency survival techniques. For us and the many people he's helped, Aton is the last word on preparedness. His methods and recommendations for gear come from years of rigorous testing and personal experience.

PREPAREDNESS NOW! provides readers with a solid preparedness plan and a glimpse into what's needed for emergencies that require more than three days for civilized life to regain normalcy.

We support a self-reliant sensibility and the strength and awareness it provides.

Jodi Wille
Adam Parfrey
Process

"Hurricane Katrina has shown us that the country is no more prepared for a terrorist attack today than it was on Sept. 11, 2001. The question is what to do with that information.

"How do we protect ourselves and our families, knowing that the government is probably not going to protect us?... Preparedness now is more important than ever."

—Sally Quinn, *Washington Post*, 9/16/05

"We don't like anticipating disasters. It suggests pessimism and America is largely a nation of optimists. But when you look at the damage inflicted by an accidental storm, you have to think about the sheer havoc that an intentional terrorist attack may produce one of these days. We want to believe that no one will ever use a weapon of mass destruction against one of our cities. But it's almost inevitable that someone, someday will. We don't like to hear that. We certainly don't want to contemplate the consequences. But we need to talk about it and we need to plan for it. The very worst thing you can do when confronting a potential disaster is to take the position that it'll never happen to us."

—Ted Koppel, *Nightline*, 8/30/05

Introduction

HOW TIME FLIES! JUST AS WE WERE PUTTING TOGETHER THE "EXTREME WEATHER" chapter of the first edition of this book, Hurricane Katrina hit. Since then, our country has had the misfortune of experiencing a wide array of disasters, from small to cataclysmic. Every single year brings with it tornados, droughts, floods, earthquakes, and crime.

You'd think that by now our system would have gotten the message and built a solid response infrastructure. But it hasn't.

We've learned quite a bit about how to respond to and mitigate disasters when they occur—but we still haven't taken the necessary measures to protect ourselves from them. Our country remains shockingly unprepared for emergencies of every type, shape, and size.

For example, our borders and ports remain porous. These conditions present potential terrorists with a relatively easy route through which they could smuggle a weapon of mass destruction directly into our largest cities. Or take the rapidly escalating drug cartel violence along the border separating Mexico and the United States, which could erupt into a full-scale war, further compromising security and stability.

Our hospitals and medical professionals still haven't been equipped with the resources they will need to handle the staggering number of injuries that could occur after a mega-disaster such as the detonation of a nuclear device, a terrorist attack against a nuclear power facility, or even a Chernobyl-type accident.

Nor are they ready for the tsunami-size wave of grief and chaos that would be created by a large-scale pandemic, a major earthquake in a densely populated city or a bio-weapon attack on a scale larger than the

2001 incidents. Consider what is written in the executive summary of a Congressional report regarding terrorism released in late 2008 titled "World at Risk." It states that:

The Commission believes that unless the world community acts decisively and with great urgency, it is more likely than not that a weapon of mass destruction will be used in a terrorist attack somewhere in the world by the end of 2013. The Commission further believes that terrorists are more likely to be able to obtain and use a biological weapon than a nuclear weapon. The Commission believes that the U.S. government needs to move more aggressively to limit the proliferation of biological weapons and reduce the prospect of a bio-terror attack.

With each day that passes, we move closer to this hypothetical situation becoming a reality.

Additionally, we have no plans to prepare for and respond to a threat called a "global geophysical event," or GGE. The Royal Society defines GGEs as "natural phenomena capable of having wholesale deleterious consequences for the world's environment, economy, and society." They could come in the form of a volcanic "super eruption," earthquake, tsunami (one significantly larger than the Indonesian event), or the impact of a large comet or asteroid.

In 2036, many astronomers believe that the Earth could be hit with a quarter-mile wide asteroid called Apophis, that would impact with the energy of 100,000 Hiroshima-size atomic bombs.

Whatever does occur, one simple fact is crystal clear. It's not a matter of *if* these calamities will happen... but *when*.

It is the intention of the enlarged and updated edition of this book to help you to be ready when these disasters do occur. When a disaster of any size strikes, you become your own first responder. If it is a large-scale event that produces extreme infrastructural damage, you may be forced to become self-reliant for long periods of time. Being well prepared will not only allow you to confront and survive disasters and emergencies, it will also help to minimize or eliminate property damage, prevent physical injury, emotional trauma, and reduce your fears and anxieties about them.

A self-reliant attitude also assists professional responders, law enforcement, and the military by allowing them to focus their attention on the most desperate and critical situations.

There is an ancient Chinese curse that says, "May you live in interesting times." I firmly believe that we are entering into the most "interesting" period in our nation's existence.

Global warming-related climate changes are beginning to take effect, while the world economy is rapidly declining. The Afghanistan conflict is escalating, along with two dozen more major and minor wars around the world. Iran may be developing nuclear weapons, the growing global water and food shortage is worsening, our environment is degrading and natural disasters are increasing in their frequency and magnitude.

This is why I firmly believe that the time has come for all of us to make the commitment to prepare ourselves. This book provides you with practical, real world, time-tested information that you can immediately apply.

The preparedness paradigm has shifted. The time has come for you to shift with it. Not yesterday, not tomorrow: PREPAREDNESS NOW!

Aton Edwards
International Preparedness Network

CHAPTER 1

Facing the Facts
and Preparing
for Them

"This increase of power from the mere musket and the little cannon all the way to the hydrogen bomb in a single lifetime is indicative of the things that have happened to us. They indicate how far the advances of science have outraced our social consciousness, how much more we have developed scientifically than we are capable of handling emotionally and intellectually."
— *Dwight D. Eisenhower*

THE MILLENNIUM ASSESSMENT REPORT, DRAFTED IN THE YEAR 2000 BY 1,360 OF THE world's top scientists and backed by the World Bank and United Nations, reports that we have polluted, exhausted or completely destroyed over two-thirds of the Earth's most critical resources, including the most important, our fresh water supply.

We continue to act as though we had a spare planet to exploit once we've torn the life from this one. But we don't. Besides doing everything we can to minimize future damage to the planet, we all must begin, in a grounded and practical way, to prepare ourselves for the consequences of our global environmental crisis.

Then there is terrorism, which, is a modern-day form of war practiced by fundamentalists of various religions and political beliefs. Some researchers have remarked that the causes and events of 9/11 are still not entirely clear. Whatever the cause, the results are evident: thousands of Americans have died, and more terrorist incidents are on their way.

Information in this book will help you develop a personal life-defense plan to protect yourself and your family from nearly anything that *Homo sapiens,* Mother Nature or the devil himself can dish out.

Destructive Weather and Natural Disasters

[Severe Storms and Floods, Hurricanes, Typhoons, Tornadoes, Droughts, Heat and Cold Waves, Earthquakes, Volcanic Eruptions, Tsunamis]

We are already beginning to see some of global warming's ominous effects, such as the melting snow cap on Mt. Kilimanjaro in Kenya, cracks in the Arctic ice shelf, and the increase in frequency and destructiveness of hurricanes, typhoons and tornadoes.

Extreme weather changes will also spread disease by altering the migratory and reproductive patterns of animals and insects. According to a report commissioned by the UK's Department of Environment, Food and Rural Affairs, climate change could soon lead to the extinction of many animals including migratory birds. Disease-carrying animals such as the deer mouse (hantavirus), rat and flea (bubonic plague), deer tick (Lyme disease), mosquito (yellow fever, malaria, encephalitis, dengue), and others will seek out new areas where they can survive, nest, multiply, and make the two-legged vermin that roam our metropolitan streets seem relatively tame in comparison.

As we have seen in New Orleans and Southeast Asia, Mother Nature may decide at any moment to show us who's boss and wash us away with tidal waves and hurricanes, rock us with earthquakes, or even blow us away with a "super volcanic eruption" as in April 1815 when Tambora in Indonesia exploded violently and an estimated 92,000 people were killed. Rare as they are, events this catastrophic need to be taken seriously.

According to BBC News (August 9, 2004), scientists have their eye on an insecure rock the size of the Isle of Man on the Canary Island of La Palma:

> The rock is in the process of slipping into the sea and Professor Bill McGuire, director of the Benfield Grieg Hazard Research Centre fears that when it finally collapses, the resulting tsunami will cause massive destruction along the coasts of countries like the USA, UK and many on the African continent within a matter of hours.
>
> The triggering factor could be the eruption of the volcano on La Palma, called Cumbre Vieja, which could feasibly blow "anytime" according to Professor McGuire.

Catastrophic global geophysical events (or gee-gee's) happen infrequently, but they do happen, and scientists are concerned that another may occur at any time. Professor Stephen Self writes in a 2005 report for the Geological Society of London that gee-gee's could "result in the devastation of world agriculture, severe disruption of food supplies, and mass starvation."

Sometime in the future, one or more of the world's largest cities, particularly along the Pacific "Ring of Fire," will likely experience a massive earthquake or volcanic eruption that will inflict enormous damage. If you live in a vulnerable city, make sure to keep a Grab-and-Go Bag at the ready. (See Chapter 4 for "Grab-and-Go Bag" information.)

Large meteor collisions have occurred, and could happen again at any time. The most recent event was in Tunguska, Russia, in 1908. Over 800 square miles of Siberian forest were flattened by the exploding object that never even hit the ground. On March 8, 2002, an 80- to 130-meter-long asteroid tagged 2002 EM7 passed within 298,400 miles of Earth—a negligible distance in astronomical terms—and it remained undetected until after it passed.

If that wasn't close enough, on March 2, 2009, a 115-foot asteroid tagged DD45 missed impacting Earth by 42,000 miles, or only twice the distance of orbiting geosynchronous satellites. It was roughly the same size as the asteroid that collided in the Tunguska region, and if it had impacted with Earth in a populated area, could have caused a staggering amount of damage. In 2029, a quarter mile-wide asteroid called Apophis will make a very close fly by, returning in 2036.

Current calculations place the odds at 1 in 45,000 that it will collide with Earth. Don't be too reassured by that calculation, because the odds can dramatically change as the asteroid passes through our "gravitational keyhole." 1 in 45,000 can just as easily flip over to 1 in 4, or 1 in 1, and we could be in for quite an interesting fireworks display come '36. Great show, but you only get to see it once.

We've also got more immediate and potentially destructive cosmic events to contend with. For example, right on cue with Mayan prophecy, in 2012 our planet will be enveloped by an enormous solar storm that could produce catastrophic problems for our power grids, communications systems, and computer networks.

In 1859, a huge solar storm called the Carrington Event (named after the British astronomer Richard Carrington) generated bursts of energy that shorted out telegraph wires and ignited fires all over the U.S. and in areas of Europe where they were in use. It also produced auroras over the Caribbean and over the Rocky Mountains that glowed so brightly that people in the area mistook the phenomenon for sunrise.

The upcoming event could eclipse the Carrington Event and create worldwide chaos, according the National Academy of Sciences. They say, "A contemporary repetition of the [1859] event would cause significantly more extensive (and possibly catastrophic) social and economic disruptions." Our communication and power grids are interconnected in such a way that a solar storm of this magnitude it could provoke a domino-effect type of failure that would wash across the planet like a huge tsunami.

Power and phone service would be cut to hundreds of millions, leading towards a huge loss of vital refrigerated medications (i.e. insulin) and foods. Transportation networks—air, rail, and sea—would be scrambled by the loss of GPS service. Even banks would be hit due to the loss of the communications, forcing many to shut down.

The NAS states, "Emergency services would be strained, and command and control might be lost." And Daniel Baker, director of the Laboratory for Atmospheric and Space Physics at the University of Colorado in Boulder, states, "Whether it is terrestrial catastrophes or extreme space weather incidents, the results can be devastating to modern societies that depend in a myriad of ways on advanced technological systems."

So… get those set belts fastened; this book will help you and your family prepare for what might be a bumpy ride.

Emerging Diseases
[Infectious Disease Outbreaks, Local Epidemics, and Pandemics]

As we continue to crowd our cities, overuse antibiotics, defrost ancient bacteria in polar ice caps with global warming, and cut down old-growth rainforests, releasing organisms dormant for eons, new microscopic and submicroscopic enemies will vex us for years to come.

SARS, bird flu (H5N1), and necrotizing fasciitis are a few of the most frightening recently emerging lethal diseases. In late 2004, the World Health Organization (WHO) released an uncharacteristically grim statement to the press that we will almost certainly face another pandemic within the next few years.

The Black Death in medieval Europe, the great American smallpox epidemic of 1775, and the Spanish Flu pandemic of 1918 killed tens of millions of people. The global AIDS crisis alone will likely kill at least 20 million people over the next decade, and as the Nobel Prize laureate Dr. Joshua Lederberg explained to me at a conference for the Society for Risk Analysis at Rockefeller University in 1995, all viruses mutate. Even the dreaded HIV could transform into an even more virulent disease if it becomes pneumonic (transmittable by air).

Of all the threats that you will learn to defend yourself against in this book, infectious disease is probably the most challenging. The strategies for staying safe in the microbe jungle take commitment and diligence. Chapter 16 provides infectious disease defensive protocols.

Weapons of Mass Destruction

[Nuclear Weapon Detonation in a Major City or Near a Chemical Refinery or Nuclear Power Plant; Dirty Bomb Detonation in a Major City, Biological Agent, or Chemical Weapon Attack]

WMD proliferation and terrorism are an explosive mix that could set off the final war that fundamentalist fanatics seem to be working full-time to provoke. Terrorists are playing for keeps, studying ways to bring down the "Great Satan," including nuclear options.

There are over 36,000 weapons in the global nuclear arsenal. The United States has about 7,400 nuclear weapons, and Russia has 8,400 ready to roll—more than enough to destroy each other many times over. The Russian weapons are less secure than the American arsenal, and vulnerable to theft.

In 1996, the Russian General Alexander Lebed warned the Central Intelligence Agency and the U.S. State-Department that over 70 Small Atomic Demolitions Kits (SADMs)—nuclear explosives designed to demolish bridges, buildings, and other structures—were missing. Most have a yield of one to three kilotons, enough to wreck and contaminate a large urban area if the device is well placed. If it were used against a nuclear power plant, a SADM could shatter the dome and destroy the reactor, forcing a flash core meltdown.

Terrorists might choose a nuclear power plant near a major city to maximize damage, chaos, and death. Or they might pick the softest target—the station with the feeblest security and safety mechanisms. Presently, there are 104 operating reactors to choose from in the United States.

Of these many targets, the Indian Point Nuclear Power Plant, which stands on the east bank of the Hudson River only 24 miles away from Manhattan, could well be a springboard for terrorist nirvana. The 1982 Calculation of Reactor Accident Consequences (CRAC-2) estimated that a meltdown of the Indian Point Unit 3 reactor would produce over 50,000 fatalities and 167,000 injuries.

We have escaped a thermonuclear holocaust at least 16 times since the atomic genie was let out of "Little Boy" and "Fat Man" at the Trinity Site in Alamogordo, New Mexico.

The first incident was the 1962 Cuban Missile Crisis. According to former Secretary of Defense Robert McNamara in Errol Morris' documentary *The Fog of War,* "At the end we lucked out. It was luck that prevented nuclear war.

We came that close to nuclear war at the end. Rational individuals—Kennedy was rational, Khrushchev was rational, Castro was rational—rational individuals came that close to total destruction of their societies, and that danger exists today."

The most terrifying instance of dumb luck came in September 1983 when Lt. Col. Stanislav Petrov detected what Soviet missile commanders feared the most: a signal that the U.S. had launched a massive nuclear attack. As his fellow soldiers prepared for a counterstrike, Lt. Col. Petrov hesitated because he doubted the integrity of the signal. Despite defying military protocol, he rode out the storm until he could confirm that there was no U.S. missile launch after all and thereby prevent Mutual Assured Destruction.

Radiological weapons or radiological dispersion devices are considered terrorist weapons designed to spread radioactive material and make its target uninhabitable. Sometimes they're called "dirty bombs" which more accurately refer to a nuclear weapon. The most dangerous form of radiological weapon would release plutonium in aerosol form. Other forms of radiological weapons include bombs, rocket shells, and ordinary explosives laced with radioactive material. The most likely targets are large cities, reservoirs, food storage and processing facilities, large transit terminals, stadiums during sporting events and concerts, large farms and financial districts.

What are the odds for further lucky breaks? The U.S. government spends billions to construct and maintain fortified military command centers—also called wartime relocation centers or COG (Continuity of Government) facilities—such as Mount Weather in Virginia, or at Raven Rock in Pennsylvania near Camp David. These shelters keep the president, his cabinet and family, and other key political, military, and industrial personnel comfortable and secure, with sophisticated command, control, communication, and defensive and offensive equipment that allow them to survive disasters. The rest of us are on our own.

Let's not forget "the poor man's atomic bomb," biological and chemical weapons, which are cheaper and more accessible than nuclear devices. The U.S. government tells us that we can expect to see both used in future attacks. Anthrax will most likely continue to be the workhorse of bio-terrorists because of its relative low cost and ease of manufacture, processing, storage, and dissemination. The 2001 anthrax attacks against five media offices and two U.S. senators showed that even a small bio-weapon attack can spread fear and chaos. A few kilograms distributed in a crowded city could kill more than one hundred thousand people, according to Dr. Lawrence M. Wein in Reuters Health. Anthrax could also contaminate large enclosed areas such as subways and office buildings for long periods, crippling transportation and commerce. Bio-terrorists can also use viruses such as smallpox, Ebola, and

Marburg. If bio-engineered viruses get into the hands of terrorists crazy enough to use them, this could radically alter the world as we know it.

According to Dr. Kanatjan Alibekov (Ken Alibeck), former head of project development for Vector Labs and the Russian Biopreperat, his former employers were working hard in the late 1980s and early 1990s to develop viral weapons. In the late 1990s, the CIA said that they had helped the Russian military destroy all of its dangerous bio-weapons, but can we believe that Russia's military hardliners did not secret away their worst man-made plagues?

Bio-warfare has also led to the insidious development of genotype and race-specific weapons. John Eldridge wrote in a 1999 issue of *Jane's Nuclear, Biological and Chemical Defence* magazine that publicly available information can be used to develop race-specific toxins and to engineer germ weapons. In South Africa during apartheid, a top-secret biological and chemical weapons warfare program, Project Coast, was headed by Dr. Wouter Basson, a cardiologist who allegedly tried to create race-specific weapons against the nonwhite population.

WMD proliferation has helped to make our troubled world even more dangerous, and unless we get it under control, real nuclear, biological, and chemical weapons, unlike the non-existent ones in Iraq, will be acquired by a terrorist organization. Then the world will see again the same horrors that suffocated soldiers in the battlefields of Europe during WWI, tormented the victims of the Tuskegee Experiment, and scorched the residents of Hiroshima and Nagasaki. I hope and pray the day never comes when you will need to apply what you learn in this book. But it might, and if it ever does, our aim is to help you survive.

Environmental Degradation

[Increased Water and Air Pollution, Leading to Higher Global Cancer Rate, Genetic Mutations, Conflicts over Fresh Water, Tainted Food Supplies]

We have overloaded our environment with toxic waste. Much of the ecosystem is contaminated with carcinogens, mutagens, and other toxins making their way into our food chain and water supply. Mutations in amphibious life around the globe are a disturbing indication of their annihilative potential.

According to the Environmental Protection Agency, over 40% of the water flowing in rivers and washing beaches across the United States is polluted. Even the underground water in aquifers is becoming tainted. More than two billion people internationally drink from water supplies so contaminated that they would fail the EPA safety standards. In countries without regulatory mechanisms, industrial pollution levels increase dramatically. In Russia, fishermen of the Ural River will not eat their catch, for fear of harmful effects of pollution. Toxic slicks in Chinese rivers led to shutdown of water supplies for millions.

In 2000, the World Resources Institute reported that "fresh water systems around the world are so environmentally degraded they are losing their ability to support human, animal and plant life. Their decline will mean increased water shortages for people and rapid population loss or extinction for many other species."

We will exhaust the earth's fresh water supply between the years 2015 and 2022, says the CIA 2005 Global Trends Report. We are also contaminating the water we have left with agricultural runoff, industrial pollutants, and even ordinary household products. U.S. Geologic Survey hydrologists found high concentrations of chemical contaminants, pharmaceutical and personal care pollutants that linger with unknown health consequences in tap water. With every sip of water, reports the EPA, we take in a soup of unknowns, possibly including chlorine, cholesterol, coprostanol (digestive by-products), pesticides, caffeine, insect repellent containing DEET, and medications such as blood thinners, antidepressants, birth control hormones, and blood-pressure medicines.

Our air is a health hazard. In the United States, three out of four people inhale air so dirty that it poses a threat to their health. In 2002, the American Lung Association in its annual state of the air report gave an F grade for air quality to almost 400 U.S. counties, 15% more than in the previous report, and including small towns as well as big cities.

To help mitigate problems from water and air pollution, see Chapter 7, on water purification, and Chapter 22, which has a section on reducing indoor air pollution.

Massive Computer System Failures and Sabotage

[Power Failures; Disruptions of Commerce, Government, and Transportation; Water-purification and Pumping Station Shutdowns; Food, Fuel, and Medicine Delivery Disruptions; Nuclear Power Plant Shutdowns; Medical Equipment Malfunctions]

We enjoy the benefits of computer technology, but most of us ignore its exponentially expanding complexity and fragility. As the global population rises, dependence on technology increases. Teeming humanity will have to manage the logistics of sharing dwindling resources by yielding ever more control to machines. As we give computers more power over us, we balance on a flimsy technological tightrope that can snap at any time.

Preparedness against these problems speaks to our need to know how humans existed in a world without electrical power and gasoline, and gives us a motivation to store food, water and explore alternative power sources.

Nuclear and Other Technological Catastrophes

[Nuclear Power Plant, Rail, and Aviation Accidents; Chemical and Oil Refinery Fires, Leaks, and Explosions; Toxic Spills; Blackouts; Water Crises; Communications and Transportation System Failures]

The Chernobyl disaster illustrated the horrific potential of nuclear accidents. Besides power plants, submarines are susceptible to accidents and attacks and are a possible source of nuclear contamination. Aging reactors are hotspots of danger around the world, and even optimally functioning ones are terrorist targets. Study Chapter 20 to prepare and protect yourself.

Civil Unrest

[Riots and Other Breakdowns of Order]

Riots can follow any of the disasters we've already considered, or they could be provoked by other causes. Being prepared for any event affecting a large number of people includes being prepared for fallout with a human face, when panic and critical scarcities foment violence. See Chapter 5 on Personal Defense.

Economic Disaster

[Economic Depression, Massive Unemployment, Scarcity, and Unrest]

This category of woes overlaps with the others—economic mayhem can be a result of terrorism or a cause of rioting. Economic disasters require special consideration because they can also arise from less obvious causes. The desperation to which the Great Depression drove Americans illustrates that our economy's fragility is another danger requiring preparedness. A massive terrorist attack, global pandemic, oil crisis, or "gee-gee" could trigger a major market crash.

Terrorism

[Terrorist Attacks by Various Means (Car Bombs, Explosive Devices, Aircraft, Sabotage, Nuclear, Biological, Chemical and Radiological Weapons, Poisons)]

The era of international conflict on the scale of World War II is over. Apart from occasional large eruptions of organized military conflict, such as that in Afghanistan and Iraq, this will likely be the century of the terrorist. Terrorist attacks are hard to predict or prevent. Their causes range from political grievances to superstitions and esoteric group delusions.

Shoko Asahara's Aum Shinrikyo cult staged sarin attacks on the Tokyo subway system in 1995 for reasons still unclear. Members of the Bhagwan Shree Rajneesh cult grew salmonella in a laboratory and poisoned salad bars, sickening hundreds in a bizarre attempt at electoral influence. The Covenant, the Sword, and the Arm of the Lord, a white-supremacist survivalist cult, acquired enough cyanide to poison major cities' water supplies, but the FBI apparently cut their plot short.

These examples show the diversity of motives and the alarming sophistication of terrorist groups, but we can't ignore lone extremists and sociopaths who may sneak past radar, as the "Alphabet Bomber," Muharem Kurbegovic, did in the '70s. This disturbed engineer, posing as a fictitious organization, Aliens of America, murdered people with bombs and threatened to release a nerve agent in Washington, DC. Aryan Nations alumnus Larry Wayne Harris, arrested in Las Vegas for possessing anthrax, also tried to buy bubonic plague samples from a Maryland culture collection.

A low-budget terrorist can make deadly explosives from commonly available materials and amplify the killing power of his or her bomb with buckshot, nails, nuts, bolts, or shards of metal and glass. Be alert for abandoned bags, boxes, radios, dolls or other potential disguises for bombs near crowds and for the nervous behavior, adrenaline sweat, and bulky clothes that may indicate a suicide bombing about to happen. Suicide bombers who penetrate crowded public places typically wear bombs that are easy for them to trigger, so you should try to put a wall between yourself and the bomber instead of trying to intervene.

Although terrorists can strike anywhere, some potential targets call for special vigilance.

- Airports and other mass-transit terminals
- Freight trains (especially those hauling chlorine, cyanide, hydrochloric acid, gasoline, methane, and other hazardous chemicals)

- Department stores and malls
- Cruise ships
- Amusement parks
- Ferries
- Bridges
- Chemical factories, refineries
- Nuclear power plants
- Water purification, storage, and pumping facilities
- Fuel storage depots
- Communication lines and satellite dishes
- National monuments
- Tunnels
- Resort hotels
- Television stations
- Nuclear weapons facilities
- Bio-weapons research laboratories
- Food irradiation facilities

As our planet becomes more crowded, terrorism will continue spreading like a disease through the disaffected. Keep your ear to the ground and collect whatever good intelligence you can find. Realistic expectations mean better preparations and a better chance to protect those you care about. Chapters 19 and 20 address terrorism.

On the New York radio station WRKS-FM in February 2001, I warned listeners about terrorists targeting the World Trade Center and to avoid the area if at all possible. My Paul Revere act saved a few lives, including close friends, my mother's, and my own. As an information junkie, I read everything that I can get my hands on, surf the Internet, listen to shortwave radio, and meet with friends in the military, law enforcement, and "low places" to stay informed about everything that passes over the bridge—and under it. As a result, I knew that terror was coming to the complex prior to 9/11. The World Trade Center might still be standing if our government had taken the threat as seriously as I did when I suggested to *New York* Magazine in 1999 that Manhattan should have surface to air missiles guarding the skyscrapers.

You've had a glimpse of some inevitable calamities. The following chapters provide ways of getting through them. First things first: if you want to stay alive, you need to be fit enough to deal with a more challenging and less convenient physical life than you're accustomed to at this time. But take it from me, the physical discomfort encountered in working out and increasing stamina and strength will pay off in spades for most every life situation.

The "Black Swan" Event

Out of all the disasters and emergencies that I describe in this book, only one truly fills my heart with dread—the "black swan event." A black swan is a large-scale, rare, and unpredictable occurrence that has long-term effects for our society, and can change the course of history. Nasim Nicholas Talib, author of the book Black Swan, believes that all major historical situations, wars, scientific, and artistic advancements and accomplishments are black swans, as were the attacks against the WTC—even if some were aware that they would take place.

I'm terribly concerned about a highly destructive black swan event developing over the next few years that will completely eclipse anything that we have experienced over the past two hundred years. It could arise from a natural disaster, or could be triggered by something human-made. I just know that we've created an extremely fragile system that could easily be unraveled, provided that the right "string" is pulled. My informed guess is that it will involve a large natural disaster that triggers a series of incidents that lead toward conflict.

CHAPTER 2

Fitness
The Foundation
for Survival

"Our growing softness, our increasing lack of physical fitness is a menace to our security."

—John F. Kennedy

THE MOST IMPORTANT ASPECT OF ANY EMERGENCY PREPAREDNESS OR SURVIVAL PROGRAM IS your physical health. Nothing else comes close. Good health is the foundation that your life depends upon, especially during disasters. Emergencies often force upon you especially drastic and stressful physical exertion.

You may be required to walk long distances, lift heavy objects, go without sleep for long periods or even live for days or weeks exposed to the elements outdoors. Being physically fit will allow you to handle these stressful and demanding possibilities much better than someone who is out-of-shape and unhealthy.

It doesn't matter what age you might be. A fit and healthy 75-year-old will be in a much better position to physically manage a disaster than an unfit 25-year-old. This rule also applies to the physically challenged. No matter who you may be, improving and maintaining your health is not an option in today's troubled times—it is a necessity.

There are other pressing reasons why you must upgrade your health. One of the most serious is our health care system, which is currently in a state of crisis and, according to a 2002 U.S. Census Bureau report, between 43.6 million Americans lack health insurance of any type whatsoever (not counting 11 million non-documented residents). This figure balloons to nearly 90 million when the underinsured are added to the list.

Another major reason to get fit is that sooner or later we will confront a large-scale pandemic. The "Spanish Flu" of 1918 killed 675,000 Americans and over 40 million worldwide. With numbers adjusted for today's population, a similar pandemic could kill 3 million Americans and 150 million worldwide. The Avian Flu is an ominous sign that suggests we may be on the verge of another.

Your health is truly your first line of defense and you must do all that you can to protect it. Besides working out and improving your nutrition, you should take a First Aid/BLS (Basic Life Saving) course at your local Red Cross to learn how to deal with minor injuries. A more seriously prepared individual would become an EMT, or Paramedic. Not only would these skills serve you during a major emergency, they would also serve your community.

Now that you know what needs to be done, it's time to get started with your program. Get your workout clothes together, throw out your junk food and fire up your iPod. I call my program "Max-3." Its aim is to maximize the three most important fitness qualities: strength, endurance, and flexibility.

My Max-3 program places a special emphasis on strength and endurance development because, as mentioned earlier, most emergencies create situations where heavy objects or even people need to be lifted, pulled and/or moved. You may even find yourself walking long distances as hundreds of thousands of people did in New York City during the 9/11 attacks.

If you ever get caught in a crisis and need to lift something heavy or walk many miles, extra strength and endurance will help you tremendously. In some extreme cases, this can make the difference between life and death. Strength training also increases bone density, important for long-term health and resistance to injury.

Like anything worthwhile, Max-3 requires discipline, focus, even discomfort. If you want it to serve you during difficult times, you must commit yourself—there are no shortcuts, and only hard work and perseverance will get you there. You will get back from it exactly what you put into it.

The only acceptable excuses for being out of shape are present or recent disability, illness or imprisonment. If you don't fit into any of these classifications, you have no excuse to be unfit.

Be honest with yourself about your state of fitness at the beginning and calibrate your initial progress accordingly; people who deceive themselves about how fit they are and what they can do can end up in intensive care. One last thing—before you begin any fitness and nutrition program, you should check with your doctor to make sure that everything is in good working order.

Those who are fit have high levels of strength, endurance, elasticity and cardiovascular efficiency. Fitness comes from engaging in vigorous physical activity for more than one hour per day, at least four times a week, and training at sufficient intensity to reach the "training heart rate." You can determine yours by subtracting your current age from 220. This is your maximum heart rate (MHR). Now take 60 percent and then 80 percent of that number to find the upper and lower ends of your target heart rate zone. When you work out, your heart rate should fall somewhere between these two numbers.

You can immediately improve fitness by increasing your level of cardiovascular activity such as walking and taking the stairs whenever possible—doing all of the physical activities that go against the modern archetype of "convenience."

Walking is the easiest fitness training method to begin with. Walking is safer and more fun if done with friends. Carry a cellphone to call for help if you run into trouble. You should also carry pepper spray or some other defensive weapon. Watch out for two- and four-legged predators and choose your route wisely, avoiding desolate places and dangerous traffic.

Before walking, take time to stretch. This is one of the most important parts of any fitness routine, because it protects against such injuries as muscle pulls and strains. Lightly jogging in place for about five minutes is an easy and safe way to get your blood flowing and muscles warmed up. Work your whole body with slow and relaxed stretches. Move through the muscle's full range of movement until a gentle resistance is felt. Hold the position for ten to 30 seconds; stop and repeat. Start with your back and legs, then stretch the smaller muscle groups. Stretch within 40 minutes of beginning vigorous physical activity. Never bounce—that increases the chances of strains or muscle pulls. After your workout, do a second, cool-down stretching routine to keep the muscles from tightening up.

The second stage of your fitness program adds aerobic capacity and muscular development. Next, add small hand weights to your walking routine. While you walk, the weights will develop muscle and increase your cardiovascular capacity. They also could serve as weapons if you run into trouble. As your fitness level increases, you can begin to add some extra movements to help develop your upper body strength.

After a month or two of steady walking with hand weights, you should be fit enough to try running. When I was in the seventh grade, I wanted to be bionic like the Six Million Dollar Man. I got up early in all types of weather to run five miles before breakfast. I would run another three miles to and from school. On some mornings, I would race the school bus to school with friends cheering me on. I became so fast that I earned the nickname "Six Million" from my classmates; some of them still call me that today. Running for an hour four times per week will bring rapid improvement in your cardiovascular system (reduced blood pressure and heart rate), aerobic capacity, and overall fitness. You will also see significant changes in your appearance Running puts more stress on your knees and joints than walking, so you will need to take extra measures to protect yourself from injury. Include more stretching exercises to help make the muscles limber before you begin to run.

If running and walking aren't your style, and you have access to a pool, swimming is the next best exercise. It works every muscle group (more than

⅔ of total body mass) and builds endurance, flexibility, and strength. It is also easy on the body because the water supports your weight and body fat helps you float. The only drawback is that you tend to use less energy swimming than in other aerobic activities.

Cycling is arguably the best physical training method of all. It works the whole circulo-respiratory system: the arms, back, wrists, and practically everything else. A good workout burns nearly 800 calories per hour and is much easier on the body than running. Even better, cycling fits into the rest of your life by being a trouble-free, efficient form of transportation. The more people use it, the better off our environment will be. The best type of bike for most people is a hybrid, designed to be used on different road surfaces. Hybrid bikes are more durable than road bikes and more comfortable than mountain bikes. For more info on bike gear, see chapter 13 on emergency transportation.

After a few months of aerobic training through walking, running, swimming and/or cycling, your next step of preparedness fitness should include weight training and calisthenics to build muscular strength and endurance.

A good home calisthenics program can build strength better than a gym with all its expensive equipment. Avoid fancy machines that turn into expensive coat hangers. Try the special exercise partner that has worked for many years for me. It's called "the floor."

You can find good instructions on calisthenics, nutrition and weight training at www.exrx.net—the "exercise prescription" megasite. There are several good books on the no-frills approach to calisthenics, including Matt Furey's *Combat Conditioning* book available only at www.mattfurey.com. This book is the best available in demonstrating how to develop the strength, flexibility and power that you may need to summon up during a disaster.

Fitness Nutrition

Proper nutrition and physical fitness work hand-in-hand. You can't have one without the other. Physical exercise will increase your body's need for nutrition, and you must choose the right foods to help it function optimally. I recommend a vegetarian or quasi-vegetarian diet supplemented with vitamins for optimal physical performance. On average, vegetarians are healthier than meat eaters. They have lower rates of heart disease, cancer, and diabetes, and lower cholesterol levels and blood pressure. They are also thinner and generally look healthier than typical flesh-eaters when they are careful to get the proper vitamins and minerals.

Vegetarianism requires few special health practices. If you eat few or no animal products, supplement your diet with vitamins, specifically B-12, D, folic acid, and calcium. Be sure to take in plenty of protein, especially during muscle-building phases of your fitness training. Learn about the prevalence of protein and other nutritional building blocks in different foods—legumes and grains, for example, are good sources of protein.

"My Butt's Too Big"

According to the Centers for Disease Control and National Institute of Health studies, obesity costs society more than smoking. The Surgeon General recently reported that nearly 30% of Americans are obese and a whopping 61% are overweight.

There are two primary causes for being overweight. Some people are born with a genetic predisposition to store instead of burn fat. If your mother and father, brother, sister or other close relatives are on the heavy side, it is safe to say that you probably carry this set of genes. You will need to work harder than a naturally lean person to keep your weight under control. If you pay careful attention to your diet and exercise regularly, you can overcome this genetic issue.

The other causes of excess poundage are poor eating habits and a lack of exercise. To avoid the disabling effects of being overweight, you must seize control of your life and accept responsibility for your actions or genetic predispositions. Do not allow talk show psychologists to transform bad habits into "eating disorders"—food addictions or other things that happen to you—you are in charge of your life.

[CHAPTER 3]

The Basics
The E-Kit and Safe Clothing

Life can be like a high-stakes card game in a crooked casino. Your success is determined by how well you play the percentages and hedge your bets. Learn as much as you can about how to protect yourself from dangers you risk encountering—and how to make realistic judgments about actual risk. The most self-assured players in the game of life learn quickly that an ounce of prevention is worth a pound of cure. Prevention is rooted in preparation, the basis of this life-defense program.

Protocols for Personal Life-Defense

The high cost of not being prepared should indicate that preparedness is worthy of your investment, even for relatively infrequent events such as extreme weather, natural disaster or a terrorist attack. I have named my preparedness and survival protocol Improvisational Adaptation (IA). IA offers dynamic and flexible survival methods that will help you to avoid, mitigate against, respond to, and recover from practically any type of disaster.

IA is modeled on the most efficient mechanisms known: the human cell and the human body. A cell functions as a self-contained unit that employs internal mechanisms such as the mitochondrion to provide it with energy, and the cell membrane for protection. Similarly, IA practitioners become self-contained autonomous units. Just as the internal organs of the human body work together to maintain homeostasis, IA practitioners use methods, tools, and skills that enable the regulation and maintenance of stability within their living environments during disasters. When individual practitioners cooperate together, a synergistic effect is produced by the combined resources and skills of the group. This amplifies their emergency response ability.

1. PREPARATION. All preparations for any disaster, crisis or emergency, begin with the individual. Learn about all of the potential threats that you may face and acquire the specific survival skills (first aid, communications, etc.) needed to properly avoid, prepare for, respond to and survive each hazard.

2. PROJECTION. List and analyze the difficult situations you may encounter during an emergency or disaster to refine a response plan.

3. INFORMATION. Increase your knowledge of emergency services available in your county, borough, parish, precinct or district. Have all emergency numbers on hand: poison control, water department, etc.

4. STORAGE. Store away and conserve water, food, and other critical materials and equipment that can assist you in avoiding, responding to, and surviving disasters and emergencies. This includes keeping comfort items such as books, music and treats to help reduce stress levels over long periods. Also learn how to maintain high levels of personal hygiene and properly store and dispose of human and other organic waste during emergencies. This will help protect you from infectious diseases transmitted by insects.

5. PREVENTIVE MEASURES. Disasters of all types (natural, technological, environmental and civil) differ in their effects, but preventative measures common to them can minimize and, in some cases, prevent damage.

6. PSYCHOLOGY. Always strive to keep a cool head in an emergency. Remain alert and well-informed at all times. Do not allow your guard to drop unless you are in a secured environment. If properly harnessed, fear can serve you well during an emergency—but you must learn to control it.

IA methods provide a solid operational foundation for your personal life-defense program. IA tips appear throughout the book to provide you with in-depth information about each specific topic.

The E-Kit and the Grab-and-Go Bag

Your personal emergency preparedness equipment begins with a small personal survival kit that I call the E-Kit. This contains critical emergency response items (flashlight, smoke escape hood, multi-tool/pocket knife, and other items). In an emergency, the E-Kit can make the difference between safety and severe injury or death. The equipment in your E-Kit must be of the highest quality you can afford. To be of any use, it should be carried with you at all times: in your purse, briefcase or backpack, or, ideally, in a sturdy pouch worn on a strong belt.

You will also need a Grab-and-Go Bag, a larger emergency preparedness bag for your home. Grab-and-Go bags contain materials and equipment that will provide you and each member of your family with a minimal three-day supply of food, water, first aid, and other important survival items. Instructions on what you need for the Grab-and-Go Bag for home, for car and for office appear in the following chapter.

The Personal Emergency Kit (E-Kit)

The E-Kit is the heart of the IA system, as it holds basic tools and simple, inexpensive materials that can help you respond to many different types of emergencies. For example, in a high-rise office building fire, if a door is jammed and blocks your escape, you may be unable to pry it open with your bare hands. Even if you do manage to break through the door, will you be able to find your way out without a good flashlight? What if you need to smash windows, cut through wire, or loosen a tight nut on a locked fire door? An E-Kit contains tools to deal with these and other life-threatening situations. It is your first line of defense against disaster.

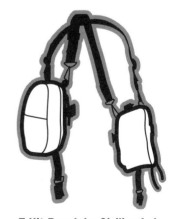

The Preparedness Checklist at the back of this book can also help you assemble the basics your E-Kit. The contents of your E-Kit will vary according to your budget and the types of emergency you are most likely to face. Even one simple tool can make a big difference. Window-washer Jan Demczur and a few others were trapped in an elevator during the World Trade Center attack of September 11, 2001, near the 50th floor in Tower 2. The men tried desperately and unsuc-

E-Kit Pouch by Civilian Lab

cessfully to kick and pry the jammed elevator door open until Demczur used his metal squeegee to widen the gap enough for the others to grip and open the doors. Then they faced a blank wall with no door to pry open. They tried to kick the wall down, but couldn't even make a crack in it. Demczur then used the squeegee to hack through two walls of thick sheetrock and make escape holes large enough for the men to fit through. They all escaped from the 50th floor about 15 minutes before the tower collapsed.

For the utmost safety, I recommend that your personal emergency kit be worn on a strong belt. It is possible for an E-Kit to be worn discreetly under clothing. If you keep it in a briefcase, shoulder bag, backpack, or anything else that can be stolen or misplaced, never leave it in an unsecured environment. An E-Kit will be of no help to you during a crisis if left at home or in the back seat of a cab. Emergencies don't wait for the convenient moment when you remember to carry your equipment.

A well-constructed E-Kit with high-quality components will range in price between $100 and $200, omitting a high-end multi-tool, E-Kit pouch and smoke escape hood. The tools should be of a simple design and construction. The following is an example of a reasonably priced, high-quality E-Kit with a good but inexpensive smoke escape hood. I've noted absolutely essential components with a star after their listings.

E-KIT

- Multi-tool, $40–up
- Flashlight, $3 (small generic waterproof flashlight)
  to $19 (Inova X-1 LED Spotlight or Streamlight 3N LED)
- Mini-pry bar or 4-way hatchet tool, $3–$8
  $60+ for Peter Atwood gear
- Civilian Lab pouch $45+
  (choose the pouch that suits your needs best)
- Pock-Its or EMT tool pouch, $16
- Whistle, $2
- Small first aid pouch, $15
- MyXcaper Personal Smoke Mask Kit, $30
- Butane lighter, $1
- One box weatherproof matches, $1
- EMT shears $2–$5
- Cord $5

TOTAL: **$163+**

HIGH END E-KIT

- Leatherman Charge ALX or Crunch, Victorinox SwissTool Spirit or RS Multi-tool, SOG Power Assist or Powerlock EOD, Gerber Diesel Multi Plier or 800 Legend and Kutmaster 91-5070CP, $40–100
- Sure Fire or Inova Flashlight, $50–$175
- Mini pry bar, 4-way hatchet tool, Beal Tool, $8–$130
- Mini-first aid kit, $40
- Whistle, $15
- iEvac Fire Escape Hood, Essex PB&R Plus 15, Technon Breath of Life, $198
- Box weatherproof matches and case, $8
- Weatherproof lighter, Brunton Helios, $60
- Civilian Lab Covert Loader, $99
- Fisher Space pen and tactical notebook, $17
- 50-lb.–test Spectra cord, $22
- Buck Knives utility shears, $25

TOTAL: **$582+**

Bargain Basement E-Kit Alternative

If your means are limited, you can put an E-Kit together for less. The easiest way to do it without skimping on quality is to make your own pouch and buy a no-frills multi-tool and inexpensive flashlight, lighter, and whistle. Stick to only primary items. A few generic multi-tools made in China are nearly as durable as their more expensive counterparts.

Taking these steps can reduce your E-Kit cost by more than half. If you really search for bargains, it can be done for less than $40.

LOW-END E-KIT

- Multi-tool $8
- Flashlight $3
- First aid kit $10
- N, P, R, 95-100 partial face respirator (in place of smoke hood) $5
- Lighter $1

TOTAL: **$27**

E-Kit Bags and Pouches

Your E-Kit bag should be constructed for durability and made of the strongest materials available. EMT pouches can serve, and are inexpensive, durable, and available at most Army and Navy surplus, and hardware stores. Nite-Ize makes a good E-Kit pouch, called the Pock-Its, that can be purchased for less than $20 at most hardware and camping stores, but you may need to purchase two Pock-Its to hold your entire E-Kit. The best E-Kit pouches available are made by a company called Civilian Lab (www.civilianlab.com). They can be worn in many different ways (shoulder harness, belt) and fitted with interchangeable attachments that increase their cargo capacity. Civilian pouches can even be worn discreetly under clothing. My favorites are the Covert Escape Trekker LT, the Specialist LT, the Scouter LT and the Traveler LT.

Arrange your gear for easy access to the most-used items (multi-tool, flashlight). The arrangement of other tools is according to their frequency of use. Rummaging through a cluttered E-Kit during a disaster is dangerous—if you have to dig, you're done. Pack the tools snugly to prevent stress on the bag.

IA TIP

To protect some of the gear in your E-Kit, purchase a retractable gear attachment system. (This is a spring-loaded device with a retractable metal line that can be attached to some of the more expensive items.) If your multi-tool or expensive flashlight ever fell out of its pouch, this little piece of equipment could save you the cost of a replacement.

Before you slide your E-Kit onto your belt, make sure your pouch's belt-loop is double stitched. If it isn't, reinforce it by sewing in extra stitches with high-strength thread. It doesn't make sense to place all that gear in a pouch that can be easily torn off during vigorous activity. It is important to note that most of these pouches are made of nylon. This fabric tends to burn and melt quickly when it is exposed to an open flame. Fire is a frequently encountered hazard during emergencies and disasters, and if you are wearing a nylon pouch (or backpack) you must be mindful that it must be kept away from the source of flame or it could ignite.

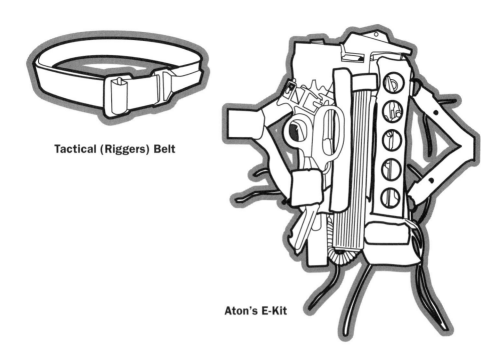

Tactical (Riggers) Belt

Aton's E-Kit

Customized E-Kits

My own personal E-Kit is designed and constructed from stainless steel mesh, neoprene, and rubber. It can be carried as a bag or worn on a belt. The belt in the illustration (see page 48) is a tactical or rigger's belt from Blackhawk Industries. My ready-for-any-emergency ensemble is topped off with a wrist piece that I designed, the Band-It.

My own personal E-Kit contains the following:

- Inova LED Spotlight and Inova Smart Bright Emergency Light
- Paratech Biel rescue tool
- Kershaw locking pliers
- Stanley mini-handsaw with wood- and metal-cutting blade
- Windproof Brunton Helios lighter
- Mini-chainsaw (for emergency cutting of tree branches)
- Sharpening stone
- Magnesium fire starter (with specially prepared tinder)
- 60-foot, 100-pound-test Spectra line
- 4 replacement batteries for Inova LED flashlight
- 3 pens, 1 Sharpie permanent marker, 1 pencil
- Pair EMT shears

- Small roll (flattened for easy fit) of duct tape
- Custom emergency sewing kit
- Safety pins of various sizes
- Modified Robo-Grip pliers
- 2 tweezers
- 10 wood nails
- Survival straw (water filtration device)
- Tube of Krazy Glue
- Weatherproof matches
- Miscellaneous hygiene items
- Technon Breath of Life
- Emergency money
- Energy bars
- Survival Straw (water purification filter)
- Aqua-Pure tablets (to kill bacteria in drinking water)

I carry a 3M 8293 P-100 particulate respirator mask and a smoke hood in a separate small pouch, along with my first-aid kit. My primary kit weighs a bit over 6 ½ pounds and is 10 ½" long, 5" wide, and 1½" inches thick. It is specifically designed for people who work in hazardous environments such as USAR (Urban Search And Rescue) personnel, EMTs, paramedics, firefighters, military operatives, etc. This type of kit (and the skills to go with it) can help you to get a handle on practically any emergency and survive in most environments. It isn't for everyone, but it certainly works for me!

Essential E-Kit Components

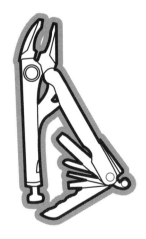

Locking Multi-Tool

MULTI-TOOL. Swiss army knives can be useful in some low-intensity situations but are not recommended. They are fragile. Multi-tools can perform a number of different standard functions, and usually include a pliers, folding knife, small saw, metal file, hole punch, Phillips screwdriver, flat-head screwdriver, wood saw, wire cutter, and sometimes inadequate little scissors. My personal favorites are the Leatherman Crunch, the SOG power assist, Victorinox SwissTool Spirit, Gerber Diesel, and the super-rugged Kutmaster. I personally prefer multi-tools with locking pliers. Even though the others mentioned don't lock, they more than make up for this function with their durability, ease of use, and extra tools. I also highly recommend the Leatherman Skeletool, Wave and XTI, the SOG Power Assist EOD, and the Vice Grip Tool Box multi-tool. I personally prefer multi-tools with locking pliers and these are two of the best around— anyone who has repaired something on the fly knows the value of a locking pliers. The Gerber Urban Legend Multiplier 700, Victorinox Swiss army Swiss Tool, SOG Power Plier, Schrade Tough Tool, Leatherman Wave, XTI and Vise-grip and Kutmaster Multi-Master are all favorites. Look for quality, not gadgetry, and don't be afraid to spend a little. During many emergencies, the multi-tool is indispensable.

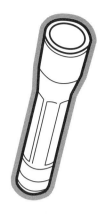

Inova Flashlight

FLASHLIGHT. Make sure that you have the highest quality to ensure reliability. My favorites are Inova, Streamlight, MityLite, Nightstar, Lightwave Forever Light, Pietzl, Sure-Fire, and LSTA. Good flashlights of this type range in price between $15 and $60. Don't forget extra bulbs and batteries.

LED flashlights are excellent survival lights that use less power than the standard types and shine for a long time, some for over 150 hours! Companies like Inova, Sure-Fire, Princeton Tec and Streamlight manufacture the highest quality LED flashlights available. They offer durable non-incendive models that can take lots of punishment, but won't hurt your wallet. Xenon bulb flashlights are brighter, but have less "burn time," meaning that they won't last as long as a comparable LED model.

Another great light is called the BoGo light (www.bogolight.com), manufactured by SunNight Solar (www.sunnightsolar.com). It is a solar powered LED flashlight unlike any other offered in the market. Not only is it a great piece of equipment, it also has a special purpose. For every light purchased, the

IA TIP

For urban environments, a non-sparking (plastic) flashlight should be used. Metal flashlights are more durable, but they are heavier and can conduct static charges that your body generates from movement. In a gas leak, for example, this could be disastrous. Make sure to buy a non-incendive (explosion-proof) flashlight. Most waterproof flashlights are explosion-safe, but you should check to be certain. If you don't mind carrying a personal survival flashlight that is a little larger than regular-sized LED lights, try a BoGo light.

company will donate a light to an impoverished community, hence the name—buy one (BO), get one (GO). It's not non-incendive or waterproof; however, it is a very bright, water-resistant rugged product that will make a great addition to your personal kit or Grab-and-Go bag.

The Freeplay Sherpa is a great hand-crank flashlight. Another such unit is made by Lentek. The great advantage here is that you will never need batteries. Drawbacks? They aren't waterproof or non-incendiary, and are susceptible to damage when dropped.

The Nightstar is a flashlight that uses the Faraday principle to produce electrical current for the LED lights. It is the best light of its type in the marketplace. The 7" RS or CS Starcore are the best suited for E-Kit lights. It is watertight, corrosion-proof and extremely durable. The only drawback to this type of light is that its strong magnet can damage iPods and television screens if you move it too close.

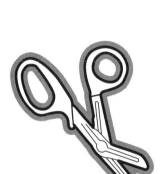

EMT Scissors

SCISSORS (EMT), $2–$15.

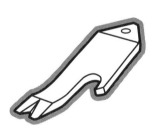

Atwood Prybaby

SMALL PRY BAR to open jammed doors, break windows, pound things, and perform many other emergency-related tasks, $6–$10 (hardware store). This is one of the most important tools in your E-Kit. I recently found the perfect mini-pry bar along with some other fantastic tools and gadgets. It is made by Peter Atwood, a talented custom knifemaker. He manufactures durable emergency mini-pry bars and other tools that can be discreetly carried. If you want to carry an elegant essential emergency tool in your E-Kit, Atwood's Prybaby, Pry Thing, or Bug Out Bar are must-have items. They cost considerably more than the standard types found in hardware stores but are finely crafted hand tools manufactured with high-grade materials.

SMALL FIRST AID KIT, $12–$30. I use first aid kits made by the company Adventure. They come in various sizes and are filled with many useful first aid items. The larger Adventure first aid kits come with a very handy book called *A Comprehensive Guide to Wilderness and Travel Medicine* by Dr. Eric Weiss, an Emergency Room physician who has a real understanding of the practical side of first aid. Dr. Weiss also designs Adventure's first aid kits to ensure quality.

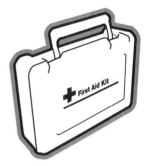

First Aid Kit

CORD. A 550-pound test paracord, monofilament fishing line, Spectra line or any other strong cord will do. Stick to a 30-foot minimum. This is usually more than enough to tie something down, or even to fish your keys out of a drain. Available at most hardware and camping stores.

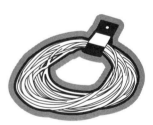

Cord

SMOKE ESCAPE HOOD. These are masks that filter smoke out of the air you breathe during a fire. The hood can provide you with enough breathable air (20 to 60 minutes) to escape. Some even protect your face from the superheated air that fires produce. This is an especially important item to own if you live or work in a high-rise or ride the subway. See Chapter 6 for more on smoke escape hoods.

LIGHTER AND MATCHES. High-end weatherproof lighters are worthwhile investments. They are readily available at camping supply and hardware stores. The best matches to carry in your

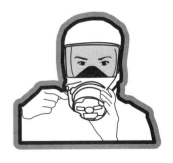

Smoke Escape Hood

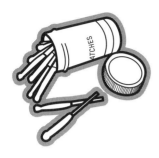

Waterproof Matches

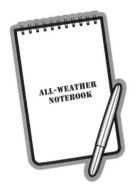

Fisher Space Pen and Tactical Note Pad

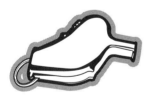

Storm Whistle

E-Kit are NATO standard-issue wind/waterproof "Lifeboat" matches. They come in their own watertight container with the striking material at the top of the cap. NATO matches have a long burn time and produce quite a hot flame. You should also rip a strip of striking material off of an old matchbook and place it inside the container just in case the top gets wet.

A tea candle is great to carry, too. Or a pack of trick birthday candles; these are great survival items that are difficult to extinguish. Note: matches or lighters should only be used in well-ventillated areas or spots that you are certain are free from gas leaks.

FISHER SPACE PEN AND NOTE PAD. You need to be able to write down critical information during emergencies—directions, first aid instructions, telephone numbers, and such. The Fisher Space Pen writes with pressurized ink at any angle. The best type of note pad is a tactical notebook, made with waterproof paper that can be written on in rain without running or blurring. Fisher Space Pens are available at most high-end stationery stores; tactical waterproof notebooks can usually be found in sporting goods stores that sell hiking, hunting and camping equipment.

WHISTLE. Used to signal for help. Storm & Windstorm plastic whistles are inexpensive and louder than the norm.

For safety's sake, include the following extra items in your E-Kit

EYE PROTECTION. Some emergencies create large fires and explosions that release toxic and irritating clouds of smoke, gas and particulates into the air. If you ever find yourself near this kind of situation, you will need something to shield your eyes. Swimmer's goggles are low-cost protection. They are airtight, durable, inexpensive and small enough to fit into your pocket.

HAND PROTECTION. During most disasters, you will be using your hands to grab, hold and move many different objects. The constant wear and tear could produce painful and potentially debilitating injuries. You should include a pair of cutoff weight-lifters or emergency worker's gloves that can provide an extra barrier of protection.

HAIR (HEAD) PROTECTION. It is always a good idea to keep a good hat to protect your hair from the elements, provide shade in the heat, warmth in the winter and a barrier against insects. Collapsible military boonie hats are great because they can be easily rolled up and stored away in a small bag or pocket.

PICTURES OF CHILDREN, SPOUSE, ETC. If your family ever becomes separated during a disaster, or your children get lost, they will be easier to find if you have pictures handy to give to the authorities. Make extra copies of pictures that show their faces clearly.

IA TIP

One of the first casualties of a disaster or other emergency is personal hygiene. Although I don't list them as necessary items, I always carry small personal hygiene items: a toothbrush, pocket wipes, a tiny bottle of liquid soap or anti-bacterial evaporating cleanser, lip balm and a few other things for scrubbing up in the field. All it takes is a few hours of heavy activity and limited access to bathrooms to go from Mr. Clean to Pepé Le Pew. Carrying these personal extras will allow you to keep yourself decent until you can settle down in a safe area. Besides protecting your lips from the elements and harmful UVA rays from the sun, lip balm also offers protection from some bio-warfare agents and radioactive particles that can be released into the atmosphere after a nuclear power plant accident or fallout from a nuclear or radiological weapon. Severely chapped lips allow for the transmission of some infectious agents, and radioactive particles can settle and imbed inside microscopic tears on the lips, creating painful sores.

E-Kit Carry Rules

Federal buildings, airports, sports arenas, and some other secured areas will not allow you to take your entire E-Kit inside. You will only be allowed to carry your flashlight, smoke escape hood, first aid kit, and some of the other smaller items. The multi-tool and the pry bar will have to be left at home, in your office, or at another safe location. When I go to Federal buildings, I leave my kit with friends who work nearby, or hide it somewhere secure close by.

Your E-Kit cannot be carried onto or worn on any commercial aircraft unless you have removed the multi-tool, EMT shears, lighter, matches, and mini-pry bar. Even a harmless item such as a smoke escape hood may raise eyebrows. Check with the airline about their rules concerning such devices before you try to board the plane.

Dress for Safety

You should learn how to dress not only to impress, but also to survive. Your garments and shoes affect your chance of survival during emergencies. When disasters such as earthquakes, hurricanes, tornadoes, or fires hit urban areas, towns, and villages, large amounts of concrete, steel, wood, glass, and other debris fall to the ground. Fires are also common during such crises. Sneakers or high heels provide little or no protection from fallen debris and sharp objects, and people wearing clothing manufactured from highly flammable petroleum-based synthetic fabrics such as rayon, polyester and nylon are far more likely to suffer severe burns than those wearing tightly woven (and tighter fitting) natural material. Because wearing the wrong clothes exposes you to more of the dangers that disasters and emergencies can produce, prepared people learn how to dress to live.

When you choose your clothing, consider six of your most important assets—your hands, eyes, and feet. An injury to any one of these (especially eyes and feet) can make it difficult or impossible to escape from danger.

Women have the highest risk of sustaining life-threatening injuries during emergencies due to clothing. The blouses, skirts, and scarves you love are often made with loosely woven, highly flammable fabrics such as rayon and polyester. But nothing puts you at a higher risk during disasters than your shoes. Twenty hours after the World Trade Center attack, I surveyed the vicinity of Ground Zero. One of the most bizarre sights was the multitude of high-heeled shoes everywhere. Women escaping the area had to kick them off to run away from the collapsing buildings.

After looking at all those discarded shoes, I began to wonder how many women didn't make it out because they had fallen or tripped on their four-inch pumps. I've heard of suffering for beauty, but risking death for it is tragic. If you cannot bear to part with your pumps, always carry a smarter pair of shoes to your job, or on a night out.

Check the material of the clothes you love before you throw them on. Some common rayon garments are so flammable, you might as well be wearing a blouse or skirt made of gasoline. Make sure you don't brush past the hot grill or birthday candles, or you might wind up spending the next few months at your local hospital's burn unit. Many women are severely burned every year in this way. Stick with fabrics such as cotton, wool, and silk, and you can't go wrong with beauty, durability and safety.

Wearing safe clothing is easier for men. Most men's clothing is made of cotton, wool, or cotton blends, all less flammable than their synthetic counterparts. But men should be aware of the smartest choice of business shoe. Shoes without traction treads on the sole are a no-no. It is easy to find great dress shoes that provide more traction and protection than your average flat shoes. If sneakers are your thing, find a pair with ankle support. Boots are the best preparedness choice, preferably with steel shanks and toes.

Both sexes also need comfortable and durable foul weather gear. Many disasters force you to spend a long time outdoors. Cheap and flimsy foul weather gear tends to fall apart under rugged use. Choose according to the climatic possibilities of the area you live in, balancing, as always, the amount you invest against the magnitude and likelihood of the bad weather.

The best rain gear is military or industrial, and made of Gore-Tex, a waterproof fabric that allows for ventilation. Ventilation is an important feature, because when they're used, rain suits can become like sauna suits, trapping perspiration and leaving your clothing soaking wet. Gore-Tex allows trapped moisture to escape while preventing rain from entering. Clothing (including footwear) with Gore-Tex costs and is worth more than regular raingear.

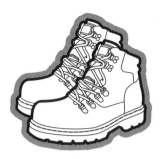

Steel-Toe Boots

PVC-coated industrial raingear is used by professionals who work long hours outdoors. This type is not quite as comfortable as Gore-Tex gear but is a bit more durable. Military ponchos are also useful; they don't keep you as dry, but they can double as a personal shelter or a tarp. A more stylish choice is the oilskin Australian outback coat, which is durable, comfortable and able to keep off heavy rains. Depending upon where you live, you may need cold weather gear. I recommend American, Canadian, German or Russian military cold weather gear.

All of the clothing and footwear described above can be purchased from Army and Navy stores or from sources listed at the end of the book. Now that you are outfitted to survive and dressed to live, you should address your Grab-and-Go needs for emergency evacuations for you and your family. The next chapter will show you how.

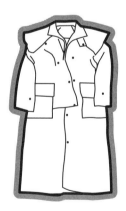

Outback Coat

CHAPTER 4

The Grab-and-Go Bag

MANY EMERGENCIES AND DISASTERS REQUIRE A RAPID EVACUATION OF YOUR HOME—OR your office. When this occurs, you need more equipment and material than can be carried in the E-Kit detailed in Chapter 3. This additional gear is stored in a large backpack called a Grab-and-Go Bag.

Combined with your E-Kit, your Grab-and-Go Bag contains everything (food, shelter, first aid, etc.) that you and your family need to survive a disaster for seven to ten days. The current 72-hour (three-day) minimum suggested by the Red Cross and Federal government is too conservative. A disaster that requires you to use a Grab-and-Go Bag will almost always extend well beyond three days. In the case of critical emergency supplies (food and medicine), it is always better to have and not need, than to need and not have.

The extra provisions will increase the weight and size of your bag, but as time passes, it will diminish in size with the consumption of the food and other items.

It is best to assemble your own Grab-and-Go Bag. Prepackaged kits are typically stuffed with substandard equipment and useless filler. The bags themselves can also be flimsy and this is not a desirable feature for something that may get knocked around quite a bit. The best thing to do is assemble your kit based on the lists below, then further customize it to fit your individual needs.

IA TIP

Buy smaller bags to place inside of the Grab-and-Go Bag to reduce clutter. Granite Gear Toughsacks are a great way to keep all your gear together and easy to access. They come in different colors so that you can easily find what you need without guessing.
Available at www.backcountry.com.

Backpacks are the best containers for Grab-and-Go Bags. You must choose a high quality bag to secure your survival materials, based on its strength and durability, storage capacity, weight and functionality.

If your bag is not waterproof (as opposed to water-resistant, meaning that the fabric provides a temporary barrier against water), a rain cover or backpack cover (available at most camping goods stores) can protect your gear. A strong large trash bag will also work in a pinch. For extra protection against moisture, "dry bags" can also be purchased. These are waterproof bags used by whitewater rafters and special forces soldiers (Navy SEALs, Green Berets). Trek makes great dry bag backpacks—a large one called the portage and a smaller model, the 2100 (available at thewaterproofstore.com). Some are quite inexpensive, such as the Crossbreed and AquaKnot dry packs. If you need a larger model, you could consider the huge Kodiak XXX bag, or the Big Black Creek waterproof backpack by Watershed. Smaller dry "stuff bags" can be purchased and used to store your food items. This will keep your food dry, and if you keep them closed tight, insect-free. (REI sells a number of small dry bags ranging from $15 to $50.)

Of the many types of backpack on the market, hikers' (expedition) backpacks are good choices for the Grab-and-Go Bag. They are designed for maximum volume, low weight, and high durability. Most modern bags of this type come with compression straps and frames, internal and external, which hold the load snugly during vigorous activity. Some newer bags come with water-storage bladders.

IA TIP

If you are single, you can use an overnight backpack for your Grab-and-Go Bag. Most high-end overnight backpacks have all the features of larger expedition bags but with less weight and lower cost. Select an overnight bag with at least 2,000 cubic inches of space. It should also have an internal frame and lots of extra lashing straps to tie gear down.

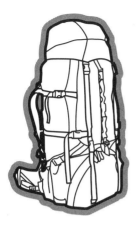

Hikers' Backpack

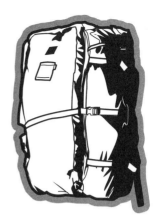

Eagle Gear War Bag

The most durable backpacks available are the ones used by the military and firefighters. If you can afford one, this is the best choice for a Grab-and-Go Bag. They are built to survive very tough conditions that exceed anything the other bags are designed to handle. They are incredibly strong, durable, and lightweight, and have many functions. Many of these backpacks have slots for ALICE (All-purpose Lightweight Individual Carrying Equipment) clips, which let you easily clip on extra gear pouches (available at military surplus stores) to hold anything from keys to radios.

My personal Grab-and-Go Bag is the "War Bag" backpack manufactured by Eagle Gear. It is specially designed to accommodate wildland firefighters. They carry lots of heavy gear into the field, are exposed to extreme conditions, and need to live outdoors for extended periods. The War Bag is roomy enough to carry everything I need to support my family for two weeks (one month if I stretch the food supply). It even has room for my four-person tent. A whole lot of bag for less than $150. Eagle Gear has other excellent wildland firefighter backpacks that can be adapted for use as Grab-and-Go Bags. The Commissioner, Mission, and Revolution bags are smaller than the War Bag but are still large enough to function as excellent Grab-and-Go bags. They have multiple large pockets to allow easy access to your critical gear and even a patented suspension system to make the bags more comfortable to wear for long periods. There is an internal pocket that can hold a 70-ounce water reservoir (bladder) and other great features. Go online to check out these bags at www.eaglegear.com.

If you are physically challenged or injured, you may not be able to use a backpack. There are alternative ways to carry your gear. You will need to use a combination of different types of bags to substitute for a larger backpack. With the right mix, you will be able to haul quite a bit of gear and supplies—not as much as in a backpack because of weight limitations, but enough to help you in an extended crisis. If you are in a wheelchair, and have enough upper body strength, your first bag should be a large messenger bag, which can be slung over the shoulder and placed on the lap for easy access to your essential items. The next bag should be a wheelchair bag. These bags have straps that can be slung around wheelchair seat posts. Smaller wheelchair pouches can be attached to wheelchair armrests or beneath the seat.

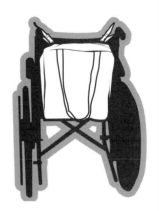

Wheelchair Bag

Grab-and-Go Bag Supplies

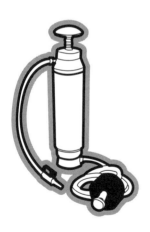

Katadyn Pocket Water Purifier

Essential Grab-and-Go Bag Items:

- Water containters, canteens, camelback jugs.
- Water (Two liters of water per person per dayif you can). 4 oz. "Lifeboat" water pouches can be used and packed away inside your kit. Be careful to keep them away from sharp objects you have inside.
- Portable water filter, purifier, or water purification tablets.
- Emergency food. Select for nutrition, weight, ease of preparation (without water or heat), ease of storage.

Emergency Food Bars are packed with nutrients, lightweight, and can sit for years. The ER Bar is one of the best emergency bars available. It comes in 2,400- and 3,600-calorie sizes and is not prepared with tropical oils that can produce severe allergic reactions during periods when medical assistance is scarce. Breakfast bars, power bars, jerky, raisins, sardines or other light canned high-protein foods are also great to include. Avoid foods that provoke thirst.

Meals Ready to Eat military food (MRE) is heavy and bulky but can also be included with food bars for variety. Freeze-dried trail food is great too, provided you have a source of clean water and heat to cook it with. Make sure to place multi-vitamins (crystal forms are best) and electrolyte replacement drink mix in the food portion of your bag. This is to ensure that you maintain the proper electrolytic and nutritional balances in your body. It will also help prevent cramping, illness and other physical maladies created by the high levels of physical exertion and stress.

- Stainless steel mess kit or outdoor cooking gear.
- Utensils: cups, forks, knives, plastic plates.
- Prescription medication, eyeglasses, and other special needs items, like contact lens solutions, and hearing aid batteries.
- Items for infants, such as formula, diapers, bottles, and pacifiers.
- Lighter(s).
- Candle lantern.
- Two Nuwick 120-hour emergency candles can also be used to heat food.
- Weatherproof matches with case: NATO lifeboat matches are best.
- Two flashlights: one large, one small, with the large one strapped to the outside of your bag for easy access. I recommend Nightstar and Sherpa flashlights, which don't need batteries. The Nightstar flashlight is best because it is much more durable, waterproof and non-incendive. I discourage choosing

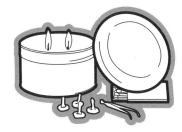

Nuwick Emergency Candles

regular battery-powered flashlights as your Grab-and-Go Bag emergency lights. You are much better off with a battery-free model. They're a bit more expensive, but you will find that they are worth every extra penny you pay when you are caught in an emergency. Batteries are difficult to come by during disasters. Choosing battery-free flashlights for your Grab-and-Go Bag is the most logical and even safest option.

Your main Grab-and-Go bag light might need to be a bit brighter than your other flashlight, as it may be used to provide light while walking through dark hazardous areas, or signaling, or even spotting someone in the dark that may be lost or injured. I suggest purchasing a hand-cranked Dynamo Spotlight. It's about five times brighter than the brightest LED flashlight, and is also surprisingly inexpensive. Thinkgeek.com offers a great model for $34.95.

IA TIP

Do not buy the inexpensive knock-off flashlights you see on TV or find on the street. They are unreliable. Only a real Nightstar will do.

- Radio: hand-crank or solar only—no battery power radios.
- Crowbar or four-way hatchet tool.
- Roll of duct tape: flatten the roll first to save space.
- 550-lb. test nylon cord.
- Insect repellent: Make sure the repellent protects against mosquitoes, ticks, sand- and horse flies, and other disease-carrying insects. If you live in an area that is infested with mosquitoes, purchase the strongest type available. If you don't want to use insect repellent you will need to carry a good mosquito net.
- Clothing detergent: a small bottle of concentrated liquid such as Tide. Can also be used as a decontamination detergent for nuclear emergencies.
- Essential toiletries: soap, shampoo, toothbrush and toothpaste, sunscreen, skin lotion, foot powder, deodorant, feminine hygiene items (for women), baby wipes in place of toilet paper. If you prefer toilet paper, flatten the roll before placing into bag—make sure it is in a sealed plastic bag to prevent moisture from destroying it. I recommend Lavelin deodorant. It is all-natural and kills odor-causing bacteria for up to two weeks with one application.

- Sleeping bag, or fleece or mylar blankets (because they are lighter and take up less space).
- Sleeping mat: inflatable or regular.
- Heavy-duty plastic garbage bags for waste disposal.
- Ziploc storage bags for waste disposal.
- Small can of Lysol or other industrial-strength disinfectant for sanitation purposes.
- Rain ponchos (lashed to the outside of your bag).
- Hats for each family member.
- Tent: size depends on number of users.
- Tarp (can be used as a tent in a pinch).
- Goggles, military style (for emergency eye protection).
- Sewing kit.
- Knife (full tang).
- Sharpening tool.
- Extra set of keys to your home and car.
- Documents: duplicates of all your most important records (insurance, will, etc.) and valued pictures.
- Money: Consider these expenses while factoring how much cash (and coins) you should have on hand, put away within the Grab-and-Go Bag:
- Average price of a plane, bus, or train ticket to an evacuation destination.
- Average price of a hotel or motel room (or rooms if you have a large family) for a minimum of three days to a maximum of two weeks.
- Average price of gas and tolls (if you drive).
- Average price of food for your entire family for two weeks.
- Miscellaneous expenses.
- First Aid Kit (see section below).

IA TIP

A good knife is an indispensable tool in an emergency, and I recommend getting the best one you can afford. A full-tang knife is constructed of one continuous piece of metal, end to end. It should be made of high-grade steel, such as tool or stainless, for protection from corrosion. Single-edged blades are sharp along the bottom edge. The top of the blade may be flat or have a serrated section. Double-edged blades, designed for combat, are not effective or desirable work tools.

If you own and include a knife in your Grab-and-Go Bag, you should also own a sharpener. A dull knife is a useless tool. The best kind of full-tang knife will include a metal pommel (cap) on the handle for pounding, serrations for cutting and will be thick enough to pry and chop with.

Ontario knives offers an inexpensive knife called the SP8 that makes a great Grab-and-Go Bag knife. It even has saw teeth on the back. An even better Grab-and-Go Bag knife is the Spetznaz Survival Machete offered only by Siegler & Co. It weighs one pound and can be used as a machete, knife, shovel, hammer, ice pick/sewing needle, saw, pry bar, ruler, navigational sight, parachute cord cutter, screwdriver, wrench and more. Before adding a knife to your E-Kit or Grab-and-Go Bag, check local carry laws.

Recommended Grab-and-Go Bag Items:

- Work gloves.
- Tri-fold shovel.
- Section of stainless steel bailing wire (used for repairs, *e.g.,* of broken glasses).
- Tube of Seam Grip (for emergency tent repair).
- Six to ten ALICE clips.
- Two signal mirrors.
- Pistol belt.
- Combat suspender.
- Portable stove (multi-fuel is best).
- Fuel and fuel bottles.
- Pack of fish hooks.
- Five assorted sinkers.
- Spool of 30-lb. test fishing line.
- Cat litter (for sanitation purposes, to be carried on your hand cart).
- Chlorophyll to reduce smell of waste material.
- Extra cotton underwear.
- Three pairs of wick-dry socks.
- Two pairs of seal socks.
- Two pairs of sorbothane shock soles.
- Extra pair of sturdy shoes (tied to the outside of the backpack).
- Two pairs of comfortable work pants.
- Non-essential toiletries: foot powder, shampoo, razors and small can of shaving lotion.
- Sunglasses.
- Powdered drink mix, tea, coffee, etc.
- Mini-folding chair.

- Magnesium fire starter.
- Safety or construction helmet. This is especially important if you live in seismically active areas. I use a military PASGT (Personnel Armor System Ground Troop) helmet as my protection. A skateboarder or bicycle helmet will work fine in a pinch.
- FRS or GMRS walkie-talkies. If you have other family members, walkie-talkies are great tools to include in your Grab-and-Go Bag.

First Aid Kit

In an emergency, basic first aid knowledge can mean the difference between life and death. If you have never had any first aid training, I recommend that you sign up at your local Red Cross or hospital for a BLS (Basic Life Saving) and first aid course.

A well-stocked First Aid Kit is essential. What you pack in your First Aid Kit should correspond with what you know about first aid—never pack what you couldn't use. Good pre-packaged family-sized First Aid Kits can be had for between $50 and $100. Adventure Medical Kits (www.adventuremedicalkits. com) makes a number of excellent First Aid Kits. You can put together a comparable kit for much less if you are willing to gather the gear and a strong bag (with belt loops or ALICE clips) to carry it. Below are items found in my own Grab-and-Go Bag First Aid Kit.

- CPR Kit.
- Band-Aids (assorted sizes).
- isopropyl alcohol (small bottle).
- Gauze pads: one each (per family member) of various size pads.
- Talcum powder (small bottle).
- Hydrogen peroxide (small bottle).
- Spenco second skin dressing kits (two per family member).
- Tincture of iodine (small bottle).
- Extra-strength Motrin (or generic version), small bottle.
- Extra-strength Tylenol (or generic version), small bottle.
- Ipecac syrup (small bottle).
- Aspirin (small bottle).
- Tube of micronazole cream.
- Bottle of mineral oil.
- Triple antibiotic cream.
- Bottle of eyewash and eye pads.
- Smelling salts.

- Large roll first aid tape (small for single people).
- Four maxi sanitary napkins (for blood absorption from deep lacerations, avulsions, and puncture wounds).
- Scalpel with extra blades.
- Two tweezers (one regular size and one small "gripper").
- Epi-pen (for anaphylaxis—for those allergic to insect stings and bites).
- Candle with a pack of weatherproof matches (to sterilize instruments).
- EMT shears.
- Lighter.
- Irrigating syringe (pump or bulb).
- Small pack of sterile cotton balls.
- Pack of sterile swabs.
- Vacuum extractor snakebite kit (if you live in a region where poisonous snakes are common).
- Rubber tourniquet.
- Ace bandages (one per family member).
- Two sterile rolls of gauze.
- Bottle of visine eye drops.
- Two thermometers (digital).
- Six pairs of latex gloves (or nitrile if you are allergic to latex).
- R,P,N-100 or 95 respirator masks: preferably rated R (resistant to) or P (partially resistant to) organic dusts and mists, one per family member.
- Bottle or pack of potassium iodate (ki) or iodide (KIO^3) for nuclear emergencies, one per family member.
- Tube of hydrocortisone.
- Small bottle of Anbesol and dental emergency kit.
- Tube of Libucaine.
- Starr Optic drops, 1–2 oz. bottle (ear pain, wax).
- Bottle or box of Pepto-Bismol or whatever you prefer for gastric relief.
- Charcoal: medical grade—keep this in your First Aid Kit.

Grab-and-Go Bag Storage

Your Grab-and-Go Bag must be stored in an area that permits easy and rapid access. Place it near a door, window, fire escape (if applicable), or other exit free of obstructions and flammable materials. Keep it away from high-risk areas such as the kitchen (prone to fire) and other potential danger areas (electrical outlets with multiple plugs, electric or gas heaters). Do not put it any other place where it is not readily accessible. You may not have time to dig if an emergency comes.

You must also take into consideration the weight of your bag. It should be no more than one-quarter of your total body weight when fully packed. If you are physically fit and very strong, you should be able to carry more. For example, in some cases, combat troops carry backpacks that weigh upwards of 80 pounds. If you are out of shape, don't even think about overpacking!

Never pack more than you can carry, or even drag for an extended period and distance. You won't do yourself or your family any good if they have to drag you to the shelter after you pass out from exhaustion, a heart attack or some other type of stress-related illness during a disaster. Know your limitations and you won't go wrong.

The cost of Grab-and-Go Bags can vary greatly. It all depends on the components that you choose and of course where you purchase them. Generally speaking, if you use high-end components, your Grab-and-Go Bag could be costly. Just realize that spending more does not necessarily get you better gear. This is all about what you need, and most importantly *what you know.* If you are on a budget, and you exercise good judgment, you can assemble a fully stocked Grab-and-Go Bag for about $250. If you really shop for bargains, you can do it for less than $200.

How to Carry Your Gear

After a nuclear accident or terrorist attack with a nuclear weapon, dirty bomb, or biological weapons, emergency shelters could be many miles away from the contaminated area. In these extreme cases, vehicular travel may be made impossible by congestion. The only practical way that you could move away from the contaminated area is by bicycle or on foot. You would need to be able to carry or pull your gear for long distances. If you need to walk, a sturdy luggage cart can help take the strain off of your back. They can be purchased for $30–$150. Many can haul up to 150 pounds (not that you would ever carry this much gear). The handiest ones fold flat. Or you could use special carts called "game haulers" used by hunters to carry their "trophies" out of the woods over rugged terrain. In the

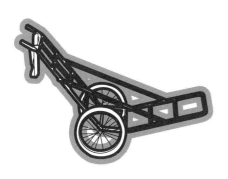

Game Hauler

military these are called ATACS (All Terrain All-Purpose Cart-Sled). Ameristep makes a fantastic backpack game cart that can be folded up and worn like a backpack. It has a 250-pound capacity and costs approximately $150; it will allow you to haul three times as much gear for long distances without straining yourself.

If you own a good bicycle, you can buy a bicycle cart and bags to haul a significant amount of gear easily.

You should regularly stage emergency evacuation drills, putting on all of the gear and leaving your home, aiming to eventually get all of your gear on and be out of your house in less than one minute.

Grab-and-Go Bags for the Office

The unexpected may very well strike while you are at work. You should have a smaller, streamlined version of the Grab-and-Go Bag to leave in your office or workspace. The office Grab-and-Go Bag should be well constructed and contain the following:

- Flashlight (non-incendive).
- Small emergency radio.
- Mini-pry bar (if you don't include it in your E-Kit).
- Energy bars.
- Small First Aid Kit.
- Emergency rain poncho.
- Smoke Hood (even if you have one in your main E-Kit).
- Bottle of water.
- Small roll of duct tape.
- 550-lb. test cord.
- Extra keys (to your home and vehicle).
- Extra medication (if needed).
- Extra glasses (sports glasses, if needed).
- Extra ID.
- Change of clothes (if possible).
- Add anything useful during an extended stay at your office or in making your way home or out of the city after a major disaster. Some of my fellow IPN members keep airline and railroad tickets in their office bags, and a few keep emergency money. Finally, you would be wise to keep a bicycle at your place of work for emergency transportation.

Grab-and-Go Bags for Your Car

Keep another version of your Grab-and-Go Bag in your car. If you attempt to leave a large city in your car during a disaster, you will spend a lot of time in seemingly endless traffic jams caused by detours, roadblocks, and similar problems. Therefore, your automobile Grab-and-Go Bag should be almost as well stocked (if not equal to) the one in your home. A good auto emergency kit will include:

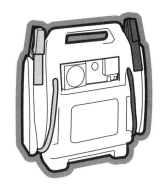

Portable Battery Charger

- Emergency battery charger.
- Photovoltaic trickle battery charger.
- Water (five gallons at least).
- Non-perishable food.
- Blankets.
- Tri-folding shovel.
- Road flares.
- Reading material, playing cards, Music CDs—whatever you prefer to do while you sit in traffic. Include a solar or hand crank-powered radio or CD player to avoid wasting valuable car battery power.
- Tidy Cat Litter, Small Trash Bags, Baby Wipes, and Empty Water Container with a Sealable Cap and…Bedpan. You are probably asking yourself, what are these last few items for? You will be in traffic for a long time. Eventually, nature will call and you will be compelled to answer. In a huge traffic jam, private spaces are not accessible; you will probably have to do it in your car. The thought is disturbing and disgusting, and I don't even like to bring it up, but I would be remiss if I didn't. If you have to evacuate a city by car, the worst thing to do is to leave your vehicle to evacuate your bowels or bladder.

    When you leave your car, you expose yourself to all of the danger and chaos on the street and increase your chances of a carjacking. If things are bad enough to prompt a large urban evacuation, you would be surprised at how fast a thief can get into your car and drive away while you urinate. You must wait until you get into a secure area where there is less traffic and confusion, or use an in-car method.

    When nature calls, a large water container (one gallon) will allow you to store away a few trips' worth of your used water. This is easier for men than for women, who should stash a small funnel and short length of tubing that fits over the neck in your glove compartment, to get the job done neatly. As for your solid waste, the best option is to stash a bedpan in your car. Throw a little Tidy Cat litter in the pan and take care of your business. I'm sure that everything will come out fine.

- ■ Car air freshener.
- ■ Road maps of your area and surrounding areas.
- ■ Extra pair of comfortable shoes and change of clothes.
- ■ Self-defense equipment (pepper spray, mace, stun or taser weapon). If you think that road rage is bad during times of peace, wait until you see what happens during a protracted disaster. You will need to carry some self-defense device to protect yourself, your family, and your vehicle.
- ■ Towing line or chain.
- ■ Small fire extinguisher mounted inside the passenger compartment.
- ■ Spare tire and jack, and non-explosive emergency flat fixer.
- ■ Soap and other toiletries.
- ■ Radio scanner (see emergency communications section).
- ■ First aid kit (full size with CPR kit).
- ■ Sturdy backpack to store away all your gear.
- ■ Add anything not on the list but needed in light of your own circumstances. You could also include emergency protective coveralls (Tyvek), another smoke escape hood, or a two-way radio. Finally, always keep your oil and other critical fluids fresh and at the right levels, and your gas tank as full as possible.

IA TIP

If you ever find yourself in this situation, it is a good idea to purchase chlorophyll tablets or liquid digestive aids. Take a tablespoon or a few pills right before you begin driving. By the time you have to go, they will have started to work. Nursing homes use this to reduce the fecal odor of their incontinent elderly patients. It wouldn't hurt you to do the same. Anyone riding in the car with you will thank you. Nature's Way makes a great product called Chlorofresh 90 SG that is available in quality health food stores.

A well-stocked Grab-and-Go Bag will provide you and your family with critical emergency supplies, food, and water. Think of it as extra insurance against the unexpected. The time and money that you take to assemble it will be repaid a thousandfold if you are ever caught in a large-scale crisis.

CHAPTER 5

Self Defense

"When civilization gets civilized again, I'll rejoin."
—*Harry Baldwin,* Panic in the Year Zero

YOUR PREPARATIONS FOR NATURAL, TECHNOLOGICAL, ENVIRONMENTAL, AND CIVIL EMERGEN-cies must also take into account the inevitable secondary effect: crime. Many people would rather not consider this upsetting eventuality, but if you plan to survive an emergency without being victimized, you must learn how to protect yourself. This is especially true if you are elderly, disabled, or a single woman with small children. Criminals almost always search for the most vulnerable targets. If you are one of the three listed, you will need to take extra measures to protect yourself, especially if you live in a high-crime area.

Another threat to consider is animal attack. After major disasters, many dogs will be abandoned. In a large city, tens of thousands of frightened, dis-oriented and hungry dogs will be roaming the streets in search of water and food. Some will be harmless family pets. Others will be strays or even guard and fighting dogs that were trained by their owners to be vicious.

Large numbers of roaming animals also significantly increase their chances of contracting one of the 11 different strains of rabies in this country.

Depending on where you live, you may need to learn how to contend with other more exotic animals that could be released or abandoned because of a disaster. In Louisiana, many flood evacuees encountered hungry alligators, coral snakes, water moccasins and other dangerous reptiles. If you live in a rural area, you might have to be especially wary of these beasts.

IA TIP

The best way to avoid the spread of rabies is to have all of your house pets (and/or livestock) vaccinated. This prevents a phenomenon called "spillover," which is when domestic animals contract the disease from the primary virus "reservoirs"—wild animals, such as raccoons, cats, woodchucks, foxes or bats.

The best way to survive any type of disaster-related street encounter intact is to have defensive/offensive protection strategies in place for each specific threat.

The most important rules of your personal protection plan are:

Avoid confrontation whenever possible. Getting into a scrap is never worth it, especially during emergencies. Don't even think about fighting unless you are forced to do so to save the life of you or your loved ones.

If the time comes when you must defend yourself from a human attacker, your objective is to *"take the person out with extreme prejudice."* Do not waste time showboating or arguing. If you are unarmed, scan your immediate area to find an improvised weapon to use against your attacker. A weapon can help you to end the fight quicker and help you escape. Never be squeamish about using force to protect your life, but be sure to develop the ability to differentiate real threats from false. You must also learn how to assess and respond to the threat with methods that increase your chances of survival and minimize your chance of injury.

When you are confronted by an attacker, your reaction must be lightning-fast. You must practice your defensive response to each specific threat (human, animal) until each one is so ingrained in your subconscious that it becomes reflexive. You can practice for this in the privacy of your own home or preferably at a martial arts school.

Always make certain to never leave your home without some form of protection during an emergency. Any cane, sturdy umbrella, or stick will do if you don't have any specialized gear.

A careful analysis of your weaknesses will inform effective response strategies for practically every situation. For example, if you are a slow runner, don't plan to escape from an attack on foot. You must compensate for your lack of speed by gaining some other edge over an attacker.

Your most valuable weapon is your mind, and one of the most potent tools in your program is deception. If you are clever enough, you can wile your way out of many situations. In the 1980s, while I was riding Manhattan's A train home at about 4 a.m., a group of thugs boarded at 59th. The A train runs express between 59th and 125th street, taking eight to ten minutes—more than enough time for a crime. I was alone in the car with them, wearing the kind of pricey shearling coat some young people in New York City were killed for. I predicted trouble as I surreptitiously observed the thugs huddling on the other side of the car. The leader, tall and thin with a narrow face like rapper Snoop Dogg's, was glancing over at me while speaking to the others. I pretended not to notice and overheard them talk about my coat and debate their mode of attack. "He's pretty big, Duane," one of them said to the leader. "We should just bum rush him." Another one said, "We should just pop the mother******." As they scanned the next car for police or witnesses, "Snoop Dogg" began to walk slowly toward me with the others slinking behind him. I braced myself for an attack.

My first thought was to take out the leader. I knew I could do it, but I also knew that I would have to fight seven others. Fighting even one good-sized person in the confined space of a subway car, let alone seven, is very difficult even with martial arts training. And they were probably armed, so I would most likely wind up getting shot, stabbed, or both. A passage from Sun Tzu's *Art of War* occurred to me: "The clever combatant imposes his will on the enemy, but does not allow the enemy's will to be imposed on him." At that moment, I figured out what to do.

I pretended to ignore the leader and his group until they stopped in front of me to ask for a light, a common ploy to distract a victim before an attack. As I turned my head up to answer, and they prepared to attack, I called out to the leader. "Duane?…Duane!"

"What's up, bro'?" The others stood there as Duane's peanut-sized brain struggled to figure out what was going on. "Damn, I thought I saw you over there, but I wasn't sure it was you!" Duane's crew were perplexed. Could it be that the person they were preparing to rob was a friend of their fearless leader? "What are you guys doing on the train this late? You comin' from the party?" This struck a chord, because back in the early 1980s, when hip-hop was getting hot and the New York party scene was even hotter, practically everybody was coming from some party somewhere in the city. Duane hesitated for a moment, then waved away his crew and stretched out his hand to give me a "soul shake."

"What's up, brother?" said Duane. I had him, but sealed the deal by asking, "Were you MCing or just coolin' out?" Rappers were called "MCs" in those days, and everybody from the 'hood thought he was one, or wished to be one. Duane, flattered to be mistaken for an MC, began to share his experiences at a party that he and his crew had attended earlier. He even told me that he hadn't recognized me at first and that he and his crew had intended to stick me up for my coat. We all laughed about that one. By the time we reached 125th Street, he was scribbling his telephone number on a matchbook that he handed me on his way out of the train. "Don't forget to call," he said. "Later!"

As the train pulled out of the station, I reflected on my close call. It was hard to believe how easy it had been to play puppet-master. A few quick words and fast thinking had turned a potentially tragic situation around, allowing me to manipulate and control Duane and his crew.

Duane is a great example of the mindset of most violent street criminals. On the attack, they are locked into a predatory mode with a narrow focus. Most are only concerned about two things: taking your money or possessions, and getting away in one piece. The quicker you turn them over, however you need to do it, the better off you will be. In some cases, however, you may be unlucky enough to encounter the more brutal type who is after more than a wallet or purse. The sadistic type of criminal gets drunk on your fear, pain, and vulnerability. To survive this type of encounter, you will need to use force properly.

For proper preparedness, it's important to learn martial arts techniques. Jiu-jitsu, boxing, krav maga, combat sambo, and judo are effective styles to give you an extra edge against an attacker. Do some investigating and find out about the most reputable schools in your area.

What Self-Defense Equipment Should I Own and Learn to Use?

This depends solely on your needs, preferences, abilities, and desires. The following is a list of the most effective self-defense tools, beginning with the simplest legal weapon that can be used against an attacker, the kubotan.

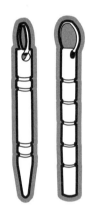

The kubotan is a miniature aluminum baton adapted for street use by Master Takayuki Kubota. It is carried on a keychain and held in a closed fist while striking an attacker, and it inflicts great pain and injury if used correctly. Again, a martial arts class is the best place to learn how to use this tool correctly, but you could practice using it on an old block of wood to get the feel of what it is like to strike someone with it. Kubotans are inexpensive and available at most martial arts and security stores. Manuals for their use are also available, *e.g., Official Kubotan Techniques* by Kubota and John G. Peters.

Kubotans

Another effective self-defense tool is pepper spray, if you know how it works and the right kind to buy. All pepper spray is manufactured from hot cayenne pepper, an inflammatory agent that can cause blindness, choking, and impaired breathing for up to 45 minutes. Its effectiveness depends on the levels of capsaicin in the oleoresin. When choosing a spray, look for a SHU (Scoville Heat Unit) number of at least two million. Practice using the pepper spray very carefully. Inert training units are available that allow you to get the feel of what it is like to spray it without exposing yourself to the real thing. The Center for Self Preservation Training (see the Sources section at the end of the book for contact info) produces an excellent training manual and video. When used properly, pepper spray of at least two million SHU can disable even the toughest attacker. The only people I have seen resist its effects were madmen and addicts high on PCP. Some brands have formulations that are effective against dogs, bears, and other animals.

There are many brands of pepper spray on the market. Fox Labs makes a very powerful spray rated 5.3 million SHU. Punch is a brand used by law-enforcement and security professionals. Mace makes a combination OC (oleo-resin capsicum, *i.e.*, hot pepper), CN (tear gas), and dye-marker spray, also an effective pepper foam spray that clings to an attacker's face.

IA TIP

When you are out on the street, carry the can of pepper spray in your hand, ready to fire. If you are attacked, the time that it takes to pull it from your belt holster, pocket, or purse can make the difference between walking away from an incident intact and winding up in a hospital bed or worse. Shomer-Tec sells a jogger's holster that allows you to carry the canister in your hand while you run or walk. If you are attacked, aim for the eyes and face.

Collapsible batons. These are steel batons that extend from 16 to 26 inches with the flick of a wrist. It can be a very effective personal defense weapon that can be used to repel an attacker or even an animal. They are inexpensive $25 to $40 and legal to purchase and carry in most states. If you decide to purchase a collapsible baton, you should either find a good martial arts instructor or law enforcement professional to teach you how to use it properly, or purchase a book or training video. Kelly McCann (AKA Jim Grover) has a very good tape called *Collapsible Baton Tactics: A Hardcore Guide to the Combative Use of the Tactical Baton* that teaches you how to get the most out of this very potent non-lethal weapon. (Available at www.securityprousa.com.)

Neck knives are miniature full-tang knives worn around the neck like pendants that can be drawn for use during violent physical encounters. Not a nice weapon but extremely effective as a close combat fighting tool. They are best used as last-resort weapons when all others have failed. This is because using a neck knife will expose you to an attacker's blood. This could place you at risk of contracting blood-related diseases like Hepatitis C or HIV.

IA TIP

Some knives are classified as illegal weapons in some places. Know the law in your area to avoid costly legal troubles.

What About Firearms?

I do not recommend the use of firearms for self-defense if you have not received extensive professional training from the military or law enforcement. Without proper preparation, carrying a gun for self-defense places you at a much higher risk of death or serious injury from an attack than if you were not carrying one. Personal attacks happen anywhere at any time, and if you are caught by surprise while carrying a gun, it could be taken away and used against you during a violent struggle. Even if it isn't, innocent bystanders will be endangered if your weapon is discharged during a struggle. Practicing at a pistol range can show you how to shoot the gun, but not how to fight with it. Shooting an attacker is completely different from aiming at a cardboard target at a pistol range. Targets don't struggle, shoot back, beg for mercy, or scream "Please don't shoot!" as live people do.

Tactical firearm training takes lots of time and discipline, and it can also be costly. Carrying a firearm legally can also be quite a hassle; permits in some places are very difficult to get. If you are not willing to go through all the trouble, don't get a gun—they are much too dangerous to take lightly. If you are not committed to becoming "born again hard," do yourself and society a favor: stay away from guns.

That said, there is no way to avoid the fact that there are staggering numbers of firearms on our streets. According to the *Journal of Firearms and Public Policy*, Americans civilians own between 238 million to 276 million guns. Over four million own fully automatic machine guns. Nearly 30,000 people in the U.S. are killed every year by firearms. Even more disturbing is that many profoundly violent criminals own firearms, and are more than willing to use them against you—especially during disasters and emergencies when conditions are strained. For these reasons, many of you may want the added protection that a firearm can provide and are ready, willing and able to do all the hard work necessary to make it a viable and effective method of protection. If you are, read on. If you are morally opposed to their use, skip ahead to the material on non-lethal weapons.

Firearms Types

There are different types of firearms. Rifles (or shoulder "long" guns) are weapons designed to be held in two hands. Pistols (revolvers, semiautomatic handguns, machine pistols and derringers) are small personal defense weapons used in one hand.

Always take your weapon to a range and try it out. Never buy a used gun for personal defense. You don't want to find out that there is something wrong with it during a moment when you need it.

For close-range personal defense, revolvers are the best choice. They are relatively easy to maintain and cannot jam, unlike automatic pistols. A pistol used for self-defense should be chosen for its power to stop an attacker in his tracks instead of merely perforating him with minor injuries that let him keep charging. Small caliber weapons such as .22s and .25s usually can't stop an attacker more than ten feet away. They won't work well against an angry large dog or other animal either, unless you hit a vital organ. You need something bigger to get the job done correctly.

My favorite pistol is the .357, for its size and versatility—many can fire two different sizes of ammo, .357 and .38. Generally speaking, I'd recommend a .38 special snub-nose revolver. Better a steel one than alloy, because the extra weight from the steel will help you control the recoil when firing. It's small enough to fit in a pocket or purse—very light, but very powerful for its size. Even someone who is untrained or of small stature can fire it. As guns go, it isn't very expensive, either.

The only drawback revolvers have is that they can only fire at most seven shots (for some special models, eight). They also take longer to load. If you want to put more "lead in the air" faster, an automatic pistol would be better to own. I believe that the 1911 model automatic is best. It was designed nearly a century ago and is still one of the most lethal handguns in the world. Battle-tested since WWI, it is still the sidearm of choice for many Special Forces soldiers. The 1911 has a strong recoil and might not be suitable for a woman or small man. But it is a reliable pistol that can quickly put down even the most crazed attacker quickly. My second choice for an automatic pistol would be a Glock. The Glock 17 has only 33 parts and nothing to unscrew. It is easy to break down and reassemble, and damn near indestructible.

Shotguns

For personal defense at home, a shotgun is best. Shotguns are much easier to use than use than pistols, because they don't need to be aimed directly at the target to hit it. This is a great advantage, because crimes tend to occur in the dark. You could also say that a shotgun has the ultimate stopping power. It is much more lethal than any handgun and perhaps more humane, because its mere presence may be enough to intimidate a criminal into changing his plans. The sound of the shell being chambered will probably scare him into a more honest profession. A shotgun is also easier to acquire than a handgun. Many large chain stores in America casually sell shotguns, so you won't have any problem finding and buying one, unless you can't pass the background check because of a criminal record.

Shotguns are cheaper than most handguns, too, but also bigger and harder to manage because of the heavy recoil. Your home shotgun should be a pump-action 12-gauge, or a 20-gauge if you are small. The smaller the gauge number, the larger the bore.

The most major drawback about owning a shotgun is that when they are fired, the buckshot spreads out in a wide field. It is recommended that you learn how to fire it properly to prevent accidentally injuring a bystander.

Non-Lethal Weapons

Modern taser weapons are a good alternative to handguns. They are highly effective and used by police around the world. The newest and best taser weapons use a powerful 18–20 watt electrical signal in a waveform that produces electro-muscular disruption. This blocks function of the central nervous system, forcing muscles to rapidly contract, instantly dropping your attacker like a rock. Taser International makes the best weapon on the market.

Old-style stun weapons are not as effective as the EMD weapons, but they can still get the job done. StunMaster offers a 625,000-volt weapon, the Stun Monster.

Stun batons are more effective than stun guns. Not only can they stun an attacker with an electrical shock, they can also serve as a club. The most effective stun batons deliver a minimum of 500,000 volts. The baton conducts a charge to prevent it from being grabbed.

If taser weapons and stun guns aren't right for you, more exotic forms of non-lethal personal defense weapons are available. The pepperball gun is a CO^2 gun similar to those used by paintball enthusiasts but loaded with pepper spray-filled balls.

Personal Protection in the Inner City

If you live in a high-crime area of any American city, you may not feel that taser and stun weapons, OC spray, or any of the more exotic self-defense devices would protect you. Criminals in high-crime areas regularly use powerful handguns to attack their victims, and they also act in groups.

Residents of the inner city encounter criminals high on crack, PCP, or other drugs that can reduce the effectiveness of some non-lethal weapons such as stun guns or certain types of OC spray. I once saw a man on angel dust shot seven times in the back and side by an angry store owner during a robbery attempt. Right after getting hit, he ran out onto the street and returned fire, killing an elderly woman walking by the store. After running a few blocks, he was shot two more times in his legs by two policemen. Amazingly, he lived after being shot seven times with a 9mm and twice with a .38 special.

To protect yourself against this type of armed attacker, consider body armor. I realize that this is a drastic step, but in certain areas, handgun violence is out of control. In some cities, such as Detroit, the death rate from firearm violence is higher than some of the world's war zones. The majority of those who live in the inner city are law-abiding, hard-working, decent people who need protection. Wearing a bullet-resistant vest in high-crime areas in disastrous times could save your life.

Legal restrictions on the ownership of bulletproof vests are designed to prevent criminals from using them in crimes. If you are a law-abiding citizen with no police record, you should be able to purchase one.

If a bulletproof vest is too extreme for you, but you want some protection, there are other options, such as a protective briefcase. These are briefcases constructed with bullet-resistant material. Bulletproof shields can also be inserted into bags, briefcases, backpacks, or anything else that needs to be armored.

Teddy Roosevelt once said that one ought to speak softly and carry a big stick. Knifemaker Pat Crawford makes a "survival staff" for strolling city streets with confidence. Although you're unlikely to need its built-in blowgun, the survival staff is an interesting and useful item. It can be used to knock

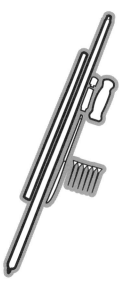

**Crawford Survival Staff
and Components**

a weapon out of an attacker's hand, push away an aggressive dog or other animal, or to help you walk through floodwaters.

One last personal protection device cannot be overlooked: a **cellular phone.** You should always carry one that is fully charged, just in case you need to call for help. If you are traveling through an unfamiliar area, make mental notes of the streets you walk on so that you can tell the police where you are, should their help be needed. Cellphones with cameras are great, because you can discreetly take pictures of the area or even of the criminal(s) and store them for later use or transmit them to someone able to help.

Your personal safety must remain a high priority during disasters. Integrate the information of this chapter into every aspect of this preparedness program. Remember, all the gear in the world won't do you any good if you can't protect it. Or yourself.

CHAPTER 6

Personal Protective Equipment
Smoke Escape Hoods
Gas Masks
Haz-Mat Gear

THIS CHAPTER DISCUSSES THE KIND OF GEAR USEFUL FOR EMERGENCIES MOST COMMONLY encountered in metropolitan areas:

■ Structural fires.
■ Blackouts.
■ Communications disruptions.
■ Transportation system failures and accidents.
■ Structural collapse.
■ Water purification and delivery systems breakdowns.
■ Civil disturbances.

We'll call this gear Personal Protective Equipment or PPE, which can also be used for less common but perilous urban emergencies:

■ Earthquakes.
■ Terrorism (conventional, nuclear, biological, chemical).
■ Technological disasters (nuclear power plant accidents, large structural fires, gas explosions).
■ Environmental disasters (disease outbreaks).

Different types of disasters share common preventive measures. A few vital items can protect you from multiple threats and hazards. It is better to own and not need PPE than to need and *not* own it. They can save your life.

Fire prevention is discussed in Chapter 15, but it serves to mention here that most people who die in fires are killed not by flame but by the inhalation of toxic smoke. If trapped by a fire, you will need an escape route, a strong flashlight, and, most importantly, a smoke escape hood.

Smoke escape hoods are worn over the head, completely covering the face and cinching around the neck. They can save your life in a fire by providing you with 20 (some up to 60) minutes of filtered, breathable air. This allows you to wait in an otherwise unsafe area for help from firefighters and police officers, or escape by otherwise impassable routes. Smoke escape hoods are must-haves for people who work in high-rise office buildings, ride subways, or are frequent flyers.

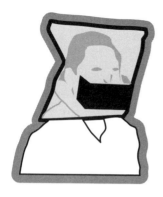

Protective Smoke Hood

There are a number of low-cost, excellent smoke escape hoods available today that I believe everyone should own and carry with them at all times. The Xcaper Smoke Hood (www.xcaper.com) and Technon Breath of Life (www.technonllc.com) models are some of the smallest and most effective available. Units such as the Essex PB&R Plus 15, $114 (www.smokehoods.com), Dräger Parat C, $229.00 (www.draeger.com), the ASE30 Safe Escape, $80.00 (www.westernsafetystore.com), or the Avon Protection NH15 CBRN (www.avon-rubber.com) are a bit more bulky and expensive, but are still light and small enough to carry every day in a small shoulder bag, backpack, or purse. They are also more durable, and offer a wider range of protection against more threats.

Your choice of smoke hood should be based on affordability and function. If you live in an area where there are frequent fires, such as Southern California, a tenement building, high rise, or any other location where fire is a major threat, you should consider investing in the best smoke hood that you can afford to buy. If it doesn't filter carbon monoxide, don't buy it.

Smoke Escape Hood Q & A

How long will a smoke escape hood work in a high-smoke fire?
Most for about 20 minutes; certain more expensive models up to 60 minutes. After the time for which they are rated expires, they become clogged and ineffective. Smoke hoods are filters designed as rapid evacuation devices. Most do not provide oxygen, but only filter air.

Can I carry it with me when I travel?
It depends on where you go. Some places, such as federal buildings, may not allow them inside. The masks are small and light. You can easily slip them into your briefcase, backpack, or purse.

How long will it last in the package?
From four to seven years. Be sure to replace all masks after the expiration date.

Where do I keep it?
If you're not carrying them on your person, keep them in well-lit areas in your home and office.

Will a smoke escape hood or mask protect me from a fire?
On some models, the mask is flame-retardant and can protect your face from superheated air, but only briefly.
Who tests them?
The National Institute for Occupational Safety and Health (NIOSH) has tested the Dräger and approved it. The emergency escape hood with the highest rating is the Avon NH15 CBRN. It was given full NIOSH approval.

Gas Masks

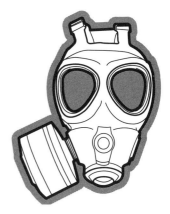

Gas masks are filters or respirators that protect the eyes, mouth, and nose from toxic gases released during intentional or unintentional disasters, a toxic waste spill or terrorist attack. A full-face gas mask offers more protection than one that only partially covers the face. The mask filter is designed to impede the ingestion of biological and chemical agents and radioactive particles (fallout). The best filters trap particles as small as .2 microns and remove up to 99.96% of harmful gas. Obtaining a gas mask is easy, but choosing the right one and using it properly requires guidance.

M95 Gas Mask

During the anthrax scares of 2001, many people rushed to buy gas masks and purchased old and useless Army surplus masks better suited for costume parties than protection. To add insult to potential injury, prices had skyrocketed ridiculously. A mask that cost less than $50 before the anthrax scare suddenly cost more than $200.

When used properly, a gas mask is the only way one can be protected from the release of certain chemical and biological agents and nuclear fallout. The levels of protection vary with types of agent used and concentration. Misuse a mask in a hazardous environment, and a gas mask could become your death mask.

If you are considering a gas mask purchase, ask yourself whether you are prepared to carry around its three-pound bulk. Then consider the benefit of a mask packed away in the closet at your home if you are exposed to fumes from a toxic spill or terrorist attack away from home.

Gas masks are designed for repeated use. They are more durable and can filter toxic substances for longer periods of time than escape hoods. Despite the brief period of time they can be used, escape hoods do have an advantage over most gas masks, as they cover and protect the entire head instead of just the face. Some escape hoods can even be used by small children. In addition, escape hoods are less bulky, lighter, and easier to use than gas masks.

Most gas masks offered as military surplus gear are not acceptable. They are old and of questionable integrity. Most gas mask filters operate by chemical activation, and sealed filters should be no more than five years old. Any U.S. gas mask you purchase should be brand new, sealed, and certified by the National Institute for Occupational Safety and Health. If you cannot verify that the mask is new, don't buy it. Beware of Russian full-face rubber masks, they tend to be faulty.

Among the many different types of gas mask, two great models are the 3M full-face 6800 or FR-M40 gas mask and the Israeli M-15 and civilian mask.

If you purchase a military mask, try to find one that accepts NATO filters. Once you have your gas mask, do not remove the canister seals before an emergency happens. Be sure to handle the canisters with care.

IA TIP

Purchase masks with drinking straws. People with respiratory problems such as asthma should know that the filters in gas masks produce resistance that requires the user to breathe three to four times harder than normal.

Gas masks for pets are a touchy subject for me, because I am an animal lover but also a realist. If you are caught in an emergency in which you need to use a smoke hood or gas mask, your pet will probably not survive. Pets cannot be taken to Red Cross evacuation shelters, decontamination areas, or emergency housing. Even so, some companies manufacture and sell PPE for pets. If you plan to suit up your pet during this kind of emergency, do not expect any shelter to allow your animal within its doors.

The lifespan of any gas mask filter depends on the wearer's breathing rate, the type of agent that the mask must scrub, air temperature, and moisture content. A standard NATO filter can effectively perform from three hours to a few days, depending on conditions during use. They can filter out many different harmful gases and aerosol mists, including chemical and biological warfare agents such as sarin and other nerve gases, mustard gas, cyanogen, arsine, phosgene, radioactive fallout, bacteria, and some viruses. They will also protect you from certain industrial gases, organic gases and vapors, inorganic gases (chlorine, hydrogen cyanide, hydrogen sulfide), and organic and inorganic acids (formic acid, sulfur dioxide, hydrogen fluoride, and hydrogen chloride).

Gas masks must not be used in fires because thick smoke quickly clogs the filters.

Gas Mask Basic Procedure

- Quickly take a deep breath, break the protective seal on the filter canister, and screw the filter onto the mask.
- Place the mask over your face.
- Exhale, blowing out all the air inside the mask out through the exhalation valve.
- A mask must fit snugly to your face to work properly. To achieve the right fit, the correct mask size must be chosen.

Gas Masks for Children

A few child-sized masks are available. The Israeli mask is the best, and the Russian mask will do if you equip it with a brand new NATO filter. Children's gas masks make regular breathing difficult, and the usual types are made for robust children aged five years and older. Smaller, weaker children need a different type of mask: Powered Air Purifying Respirators (PAPR).

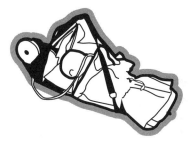

Neoterik PAPR Baby Hood

A PAPR is a positive motorized SCUBA system that blows fresh air into a hood placed over an infant's or small child's head. Coverall tents (Baby Rangers) are another option for infants. Israeli children's masks are sold on the Internet for $150–$200. Make sure that the mask is still packed in its plastic wrapping and that the canisters are sealed with a small plastic tab on the filter lid and an aluminum seal on the bottom of the canister. If the mask is not new, it should not be used.

Haz-Mat Gear

Apart from gas masks, another must-have for protecting yourself in a contaminated environment is coverall clothing, haz-mat (hazardous materials) gear designed to insulate the wearer from dangerous chemicals, organisms, and other contaminants. Haz-mat suits have different protective levels and types: A, B, C, and D. Type A gear provides the wearer with the highest levels of protection from multiple types of threat. In many ways, type A haz-mat suits resemble space suits. Think of *The Andromeda Strain,* and you'll get the picture.

Like a space suit, haz-mat suits can have their own portable oxygen supply, or be tethered to an oxygen pump. The amount of protection haz-mat suits provide is dependent on the suit's material, the agent or substance that they are exposed to, ambient conditions, and duration of use.

Over time, certain chemicals (or intense activity or conditions) can corrode or stress the fabric, compromising the suit's integrity. If the suit cracks, small amounts of the toxic substances can become suspended in the surrounding air leak inside. The time this takes to happen is called the "average breakthrough time," and the amount of substance that leaks inside is the "minimum detectable permeation."

For basic preparedness, purchase a haz-mat suit that's hooded and relatively non-permeable, like a good raincoat or waterproof coverall, one you could wear over your regular clothes to move quickly through a contaminated area. Make sure the coat is made from vinyl-covered fabric or vulcanized rubber (rubber-coated fabric). To complete your suit, add chemical-resistant gloves (this could be a pair of latex dishwashing gloves), a good pair of work boots or rubber galoshes, and duct or gaffers tape to seal the gaps around your wrists and ankles. This type of low-budget haz-mat suit is more than enough to get you out of a minimally contaminated area safely.

When you put on the suit, slide the sleeves over the ends of your gloves and wrap your wrists with duct tape, forming a seal. Repeat this procedure at your ankles and waist. Cover your head with the hood and draw the string tight around your face and the mask.

Once you put the suit on, do not remove it until you leave the contaminated zone. When you arrive at your destination, you will need assistance to remove your improvised hot suit to avoid contact with the toxic agent. It must be cleansed or disinfected, carefully cut off, and discarded safely.

Cover any gear you will be carrying through a contaminated area. Large heavy-duty trash bags work well if you double up the bags and carefully seal them with duct tape. Protect the bags from punctures and abrasions and maintain a seal, or your equipment and supplies will become contaminated. If you go to a decontamination center, you will be likely hosed down with detergent, and your clothes will be removed and destroyed. Whatever you carry with you will undergo the same process. If you want to keep it, pack it correctly.

Finally, before you are sealed inside your hot suit, take preparative measures regarding bodily functions. Depends or other incontinents' undergarments can help you deal with the consequences of nature's call or fear's grip.

Select (or make) the best personal protective equipment and materials you can afford. In an emergency or disaster, your life may depend upon your choices.

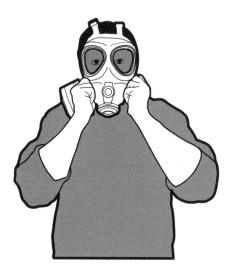

Step 1 Put on Gas Mask

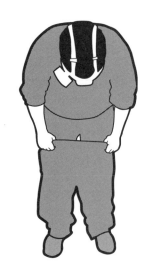

Step 2 Put on Protective Pants

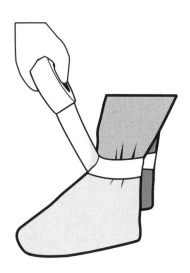

**Step 3 Slip on "Sock Booties" and
Duct Tape over Protective Pants**

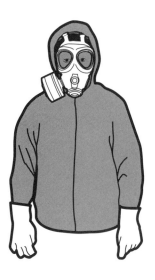

**Step 4 Put on Protective Jacket
with Hood and Gloves**

How to Put on a Haz-Mat Suit

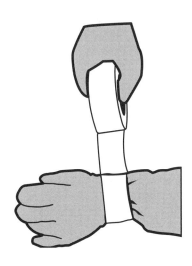

**Step 5 Duct Tape Jacket
Sleeves over Gloves**

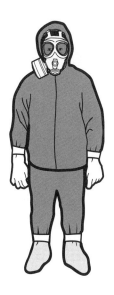

Process Complete

CHAPTER 7

Water

"Water is the only drink for a wise man."
—*Henry David Thoreau*

WATER IS SECOND ONLY TO AIR IN IMPORTANCE FOR SURVIVAL, AND EMERGENCY PREPARED-
ness includes knowing how to store, manage and purify it to ride out disasters
and protect yourself from waterborne diseases and toxins.

A natural disaster can cause breaks in water mains that contaminate water,
making it unsafe for both drinking and cleaning. Our public water infrastructure
is also vulnerable to terrorism. In 2002, the FBI warned of imminent terrorist
attacks against critical American infrastructural targets, including water treatment facilities. Don't wait for a water-threatening emergency to start a water
safety and storage program. Do it now, and you will be glad you did.

Water Storage for the Home

For general emergency preparedness, it is critical to maintain and store at
minimum a 72-hour household supply of emergency water. I recommend that
you store three gallons per person per day, for drinking, personal hygiene and
cooking. You could get by with one to two gallons a day per person, but I advise
storing three gallons per person per day, especially if you have small children
or someone ill or elderly living in your home.

Water can be stored in a several different ways. In my home, I have two
55-gallon stainless steel water tanks, one 60-gallon aquamat and four five-
gallon transportable water tanks. We always have a standing emergency water
supply of between 170 to nearly 200 gallons. This amount, reflects my own
predilection for worst-case scenario preparedness.

Some emergency manuals recommend that you buy bottled water for your emergency home supply, store it in a cool, dark place, and replace it once a year. Many people purchase bottled water as a presumably cleaner and safer alternative to tap water, but you should be aware that in many cases it isn't. There are health consequences related to PVC, a type of plastic used for many containers. Plastic containers identify the type of plastic with a recycling mark, a number surrounded by a triangle with arrows. PVC is number 3 plastic. Other plastic containers best avoided for medical reasons are number 6 (styrofoam) and number 7, which is fortunately not commonly used. Even food-grade plastic is not as stable as stainless steel and tends to "outgas," that is, leach some of the material into the water in the form of vapor. This can be minimized by placing plastic water containers in a cool, dark place, if you do indeed have such a place in your home. It is still not advised that people leave their water standing for six months. Still, people should not keep their emergency supplies standing in plastic containers for more than six months.

Whether your water is prepackaged or home-purified, it should be cycled consistently to avoid stagnation and the outgassing of hazardous material into the water. This is especially true if you live in a hot climate or if the containers are exposed to sunlight. I get my water from Poland Springs in five-gallon bottles, pour it into my storage containers and rotate it constantly. It sounds like work, but as a habit takes very little of my time.

Water Storage Containers

Barrels, Plastic and Metal

Plastic water storage containers vary in size and shape. They should all be made of FDA food-grade plastic. Never store water in containers that have been used for anything else other than water. Do not place the containers near areas with toxic substances. The fumes can leach into the containers and contaminate your water. If you are purifying your water with bleach, remember that chlorine is a caustic agent and shouldn't be used in a plastic container. Glass bottles avoid this problem, but are too fragile for safe storage in a cramped space such as a closet. Glass containers are also heavier than plastic containers.

Stainless steel containers are my personal choice of water storage container. They keep my water tasting great and most importantly, I don't need to worry about mutagenic chemicals leaching into my *aqua pura*. In a stainless steel tank, water can be stored for long periods without fear. The container must be brand new, never used to store gas, paint thinner, or any other toxic substance. Water stored in stainless steel should be untreated, because chlorine is corrosive.

A drawback with stainless steel tanks is their price. Plastic is less than half the cost. If you can't afford the extra ducats, the plastic containers will be fine as long as you cycle your water frequently and keep it cool and dark.

If you choose large water barrels as your storage containers, you will also need to purchase a small hand-operated siphon pump to draw out the water, and a bung wrench to open and close the barrels. Rotation with this storage method is simple. Since the water is pumped out, it is as easy as turning on a faucet and filling up a water bottle a gallon at a time. If you own a 55-gallon water tank and drink one gallon of water a day, you will have completely cycled through your emergency water supply in less than two months.

If you live in a small apartment, it's best to use smaller 20-gallon barrels or square five-gallon containers that can be stacked and stored in closets.

Water Mats

Also useful are water mats that can be stored under a bed. Water mats called Aquaflex Aquatanks (available at www.aquaflex.net) come in 60- and 150-gallon-plus sizes. A water mat is easily stored under a bed. If you decide to purchase a water mat, you need to understand the following:

Once filled, a 60-gallon mat weighs 480 pounds and would be difficult to move. Fill it up in the area where you will keep it or you will have to drag it there with difficulty. Place a heavy tarp underneath to prevent scratches or punctures and remove all sharp objects in its path if you drag it to its destination. If you place a mat under a bed, make sure there are no protruding springs or jagged pieces of metal that can poke holes while you are lying down or having fun on top of your bed. If you have a cat (or a dog that chews), use water barrels. If a frisky feline gets acquainted with your mat, you may return to your home one day and find your place waterlogged.

Outdoor Emergency Water Sources

If you need to find water outside your home, you can use the following sources. Be sure to purify the water according to the instructions later in this chapter before drinking it.

- Rainwater
- Streams, rivers and other moving bodies of water
- Ponds and lakes
- Natural springs
- Wells

Avoid water with floating material, an odor or dark color. Only use saltwater if you distill it first. You should never drink floodwater.

Hidden Water Sources in Your Home

If a disaster catches you without a stored supply of clean water, you can use the water in your hot-water tank, pipes and ice cubes. As a last resort, you can use water in the reservoir tank of your toilet (not the bowl).

To use the water in your pipes, let air into the plumbing by turning on the faucet in your house to its highest level. A small amount of water will trickle out. Then obtain water from the lowest faucet in the house.

To use the water in your hot-water tank, be sure the electricity or gas is off, and open the drain at the bottom of the tank. Start the water flowing by turning off the water intake valve and turning on a hot-water faucet. Do not turn on the gas or electricity when the tank is empty.

> ### IA TIP
>
> Do you know the location of your incoming water valve? You'll need to shut it off to stop contaminated water from entering your home if you hear reports of broken water or sewage lines.

Water Treatment Methods

In troubled times, the only sure method for water quality is to master water treatment methods with your own home equipment. Below are various methods. No single method is perfect, but each has its benefits. Keep in mind that if you store purified water, the chlorine has been removed, which can enable microbial growth if this water is placed in containers that are not extremely clean.

PURIFICATION METHOD	Removes Microbes	Removes Volatile Organic Compounds	Removes Mercury, Lead and PCBs	Removes Chlorine
Boiling	✓			
Chemical Methods	✓			
Distillation	✓	✓		
Reverse Osmosis	✓	✓	✓	
Glass, Ceramic and Carbon Filtration		✓	✓	✓

Boiling

You can destroy waterborne pathogenic organisms by sustaining a rolling boil for at least five minutes (add a minute for each 1000 feet above sea level). As the water cools, make sure to cover it and keep it away from foreign objects (*e.g.*, cooking utensils, pot holders) that may bear contaminants. Aerating the water by pouring it back and forth between two containers will improve its taste.

Chemical Methods

Chemical disinfection is another relatively simple, effective, and inexpensive method of rendering water potable. Its main drawbacks are unpleasant taste and ineffectiveness against protozoan cysts such as Cryptosporidium.

Clorox or other chlorine bleach can be used as a water purifier in emergencies. Use no more than 12 drops per gallon, and after adding the bleach,

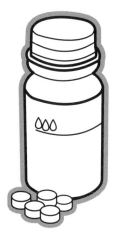

Potable Aqua Water Purification Tablets

let the water stand for 30-45 minutes. Before using the water, see that it has a faint chlorinated odor. Remember to sterilize the second container before beginning this process. You might want to have some sweetened powdered drink mix on hand to cover the bad taste.

Water purification tablets are not recommended for extended use but are helpful in some situations. Potable Aqua tablets (Globuline-Tetraglycine hydroperiodide) are a popular water purification pill. Four tablets will purify one gallon of water in about an hour. If the water is murky or very cold, you will need an additional half-hour.

Iodine crystals also purify water. Place six to eight grams of USP-grade iodine crystals in a one-ounce glass bottle. Add water to dissolve the crystals (shake softly), then add the solution to one quart of water. Temperature variations will produce changes in the purification solution's concentration.

Halazone tablets can also be used. You will need at least 20 tablets to purify one gallon of water. Once the tablets are dissolved, let the water sit for at least 30 minutes. Defective tablets have a pungent odor.

Distillation

In distillation, water is converted into steam and passed through a series of tubes where it condenses, stripped of contaminants. Various home distillers are available on the web.

Reverse Osmosis Systems

Reverse osmosis is another method of water purification that uses the water pressure in your home to force the tap water through a semi-permeable membrane that filters and washes out different contaminants. Filters manufactured by PUR, Brita, and others are quality products that filter many different types of contaminants to improve the taste and appearance of water. They are not regulated or tested by the federal government and should not be considered a replacement for more sophisticated methods of water treatment. They are good for removing heavy metals like lead but may not work against other lighter contaminants like pesticides and some volatile organic compounds. They also waste lots of water. If you live in a drought-plagued area this may not work well for you.

UV Water Purification Systems

Ultraviolet water purification systems utilize special glow lamps that generate a form of UV radiation that is much stronger than regular sunlight. This produces a wavelength of 254 nanometers that is highly destructive to germs called UV-C, sometimes referred to as "germicidal UV." UV purification systems have several different types of filtration systems that capture VOC chemicals (chlorine) and many other contaminating substances.

UV home water treatment systems are some of the most effective available, provided that you have emergency power available for them to operate during power outages. They use light energy to destroy harmful microorganisms, without utilizing any chemicals or silver. These can change the water's taste. They are often less expensive than their mechanical counterparts, and are easy to operate and maintain.

Filtration

There are many different types of filtration devices. If you are using a filter that does not eliminate biological and chemical contaminants, boiling water is still necessary. Most filtration devices do not kill microbes. Carbon filters can even become a breeding ground for dangerous microbes—because of this, you should not use carbon filters for purification of questionable water unless the water has been boiled first to fill microbes.

IA TIP

The EPA recommends that people flush pipes by letting the water run for at least two minutes before drinking water from the tap. Always use cold water for drinking and cooking; concentrations of lead and other toxins are higher in hot water. People who live in large apartment complexes and old tenement buildings must pay particularly close attention to their tap water. Many older buildings have plumbing with lead-based solder at the joints.

Glass fiber filters are woven to form pores. The fibers strain out waste and let the clean water through. Brushing or washing can clean glass fiber filters, but they will eventually clog up. Ceramic filters are cylinders with pores significantly smaller than those in glass fiber filters. They also last longer, and can be easily cleaned. Carbon filters come in granular or block form. The Brita water filtration system is a popular carbon water filter. Impurities stick to the carbon surface in a process called "absorption." Carbon-filter treated water tastes best, but when the filter reaches its absorption limit, the absorbed material can be released back into your drinking water.

Multi-stage filters combine different types of filter elements in one unit, *e.g.,* glass fiber-wrapped carbon core, pleated glass fiber, or silver-permeated ceramic with carbon (the ceramic element traps pollutants, and the silver eliminates bacterial growth by killing microorganisms trapped in the filter, while the carbon removes chemicals and improves the taste).

CHAPTER 8

Food

There's no way to overstate the value of an emergency food supply.

I BELIEVE THAT EZRA TAFT BENSON, THE FORMER U.S. SECRETARY OF AGRICULTURE (UNDER Eisenhower) and president of the Mormon Church, said it best when he made this statement regarding food storage:

> *"The revelation to produce and store food may be as essential to our temporal welfare today as boarding the ark was to the people in the days of Noah."*

No truer words have ever been spoken on this subject. You may not be a Mormon, or of any faith or persuasion, but don't doubt or dismiss the wisdom of his statement because of his beliefs. Major disasters, civil emergencies, and other crises can sometimes limit access to (or completely cut off) food deliveries for protracted periods. In some extreme cases, this can continue for weeks or even months.

Power outages and utility shutdowns are also quite common during disasters. When they occur, this will prevent you from refrigerating and cooking your food.

In light of the many different challenges we will be facing over the next few decades, it is imperative that you create and maintain an emergency food supply in your home or apartment.

The questions you should be asking yourself about the subject are:

- How much food should I store away?
- What type of food is best for an emergency food supply?
- Where should it be stored, and how do I do it properly?
- How long can the food last, and remain fresh and edible?
- How much will it cost to get an emergency food supply together?

The following information will help you build a custom emergency food supply for your home or apartment. Once completed, it will provide you with the sustenance you'll need if you ever find yourself in a situation where your access to food is disrupted or cut off due to a disaster or emergency.

Emergency Food Supply (EFS) Size

Your emergency food supply must be large enough to provide you (and your family members) with enough nutrition for a very basic minimum of two weeks. Let me stress that I'd prefer something much larger (three months, one season, or even a whole year), but realize the limitations of our cramped urban living spaces and, in the failing economy, your wallets. If you have the means, spare no expense—if you don't, just do the best you can. Whatever you put together will always be better than absolutely nothing.

If you live in a private home, you'll have a lot more space available to set up a food storage area in a small food pantry or locker.

EFS Types

Your emergency food supply should for the most part be comprised of food that requires the least amount of preparation and highest levels of nutrition possible, durable packaging, and essential vitamins and energy.

In terms of durability, canned food is best. Packaged food is also good if it is in sealed waterproof plastic. If it isn't, it could be ruined if you were in a flood or rainstorm. If you choose packaged food, you'll need to make certain to place it in sealable plastic bags. Make sure to press out as much air as possible to minimize condensation inside of the bag and decrease the size for storage purposes. If you have an infant, you will also need to include baby food, formula, and other specialized nutritional supplements in your supply.

Dehydrated Food

Dehydrated emergency food supplies can last much longer than regular store-bought products. In temperature-controlled environments, many dehydrated foods can last up to five years and, for some, 20 or more. Dehydrated foods have many advantages over regular store-bought groceries. They take up much less space and are easy to prepare, after adding water, seasoning, and some cooking (most dehydrated foods require this). Pound for pound, they're also more economical.

Best of all, dehydrated foods can last from eight months to three years after the can is opened (provided it is resealed with an airtight plastic lid), without refrigeration.

Another method to ensure freshness would be to remove the food with a ladle or large spoon. If it is poured out, a great deal can be exposed to air and moisture. Some products are packed with nitrogen gas (a stabilizing agent). When poured, the protective inert gas can be lost. In the long term, this can reduce the food's shelf life.

The only drawback to dehydrated foods is that they don't contain spices or flavoring. You must add your own, so if you plan to use it, make certain to include a wheel spice rack in your pantry to have plenty of herbs and spices on hand to give your dehydrated food some extra flavor.

Dehydrated Food Companies

My choice for dehydrated food is Nitro-Pak (www.nitro-pak.com).

IA TIP

When you choose to store moisture-sensitive dry food, I would suggest purchasing a desiccant. This is material that can absorb moisture from the air (hygroscopic). You can find it in stores that have flower supplies—or, if you want to go hardcore, dry out a piece of wood (use a heat gun oven) and place it inside of the storage medium (container, bag, etc.). Do it quickly, as it begins to soak up moisture in the air as soon as you are done drying it.

DEHYDRATING FOOD AT HOME

It isn't necessary to purchase pre-prepared food. You can always dehydrate and prepare your own at home. Food dehydration is an ancient practice that has tremendous value, and I would encourage you to learn how to do it even if you don't plan to use it to build your emergency food supply. It is very important that you have the skill, just in case you find yourself in a position where you will need to do it.

Dehydration Basics

To begin, you must use fresh fruit, vegetables, or anything else that you wish to dehydrate. Wash it and pre-prepare it in the form that you will be eating it. Make certain that the pieces of food that you cut are even in size and shape. The thinner you cut them, the faster they will dry. Before the drying process begins, add a little lemon juice to the vegetable, or use a steamer, to prevent them from becoming too tough during the drying process.

Your food can be dried in an oven set at the lowest temperatures, ranging between 130–140° F. The oven door must be kept open to maintain air circulation. The food is dry when it has a leathery texture, and bendable when cooled or, in the case of some foods, can also take on cookie-like properties and easily be broken up.

In the case of fruit, you need to allow time for a process called conditioning. This balances the remaining moisture content and reduces the risk of mold and bacterial growth. To accomplish this, you will need to take the dried fruit (after it has completely cooled), and place it in sealed containers, packed loosely for about one week to a maximum of 12 days. Make sure to shake the container daily to prevent the pieces from sticking together.

While packed, the pieces with extra moisture will transfer it to other dryer sections, balancing off the moisture content of the whole.

Make sure your dried food is packed away in sealed containers when it has completely cooled. If it is still warm, condensation can develop that can promote mold growth. When stored properly, home-dehydrated food can last between six months to a year.

There are a number of high-quality food dehydrators on the market. My favorite is called the hanging food pantry. I like it because it's non-electric, inexpensive, and easy to use. It's available on Amazon.com for $59.95. I also believe that you can't go wrong with the Excalibur ED-2400 four-tray model, or the nine-tray unit (if you'd prefer a larger unit) along with some others manufactured by Nesco (the Gardenmaster is one of the best available) and an electric model by L'Equip. There are many other types and sizes of dehydrator available. Do some research to see what fits your needs best.

Freeze-Dried

Freeze-dried foods come pre-prepared as an "entrée" (like TV dinners) and are pre-cooked, specially designed for campers and hikers. They cost between $4–6 per meal. A bit expensive, but they make up for the cost due to ease of preparation, weight, and taste. It can also be stored away for much longer than its dehydrated counterparts.

All you need to do to use them is to measure out the portions and place it into hot water (165° F to boiling).

Although most of the hardcore survivalists have freeze-dried supplies, I have a mixture of freeze-dried and dehydrated. It's up to you what you choose to use in your pantry; just make sure not to skimp on quality because of price.

The following is a list of a few products that I regularly use and enjoy. They are in my Grab-and-Go bag and emergency food pantry, and are top-grade, nutritious, and taste great. If I ever had to hunker down after an emergency for an extended period, this is the food I'd like to eat. They're easy to prepare and store, and are highly cost-effective. I can't recommend them enough.

- Mountain House (www.mountainhouse.com). They also have a "flameless heating" kit that can heat up Mountain House food. Very useful.
- Richmoor Foods (www.richmoor.com)
- Alpine Aire (www.alpineaire.com)

If you can afford it, you might want to purchase in bulk. Many companies that manufacture freeze-dried food have packages that contain enough food to supply your needs for up to a year.

Alpine Aire features a special SuperPak system that can supply two adults for one year, or one adult for two years. The 2009 cost is $7,751.08.

Mountain House has a package called the Ultimate-Pack II that contains one year's supply of food for one person for $4,275.00. They also have a four-person, three-month "Dinner Entree-Pak" that makes a great three-month food supply (if you don't mind eating entrées all the time). This costs $1,190.00.

If that's a bit too pricy, you can always go low-budget/high-quality with improvised freeze-dried type meals of your own. Knorr-Lipton has special meals called "Lipton Sides" that are quite tasty. You simply add water, or a mixture of water and powdered milk and oil (if you have it), bring it to a boil, and you're done. They have a nice variety, including treats like Teriyaki Noodles and Cheesy Cheddar Noodles, to name a few. They're a bit salty, but taste pretty good—especially if you add some canned salmon or tuna. This also stretches the meal and adds extra protein.

Best of all, you can get them for about $2 per pack—significantly less than the other meals. Quite a bargain if you do the math. One month's worth of meals for four people: three meals per day at $2 per person = $24 per day, $720 per month. Lots of money saved!

The only major drawback is that they require extra energy to prepare.

Meals Ready-to-Eat (MRE)

MREs are pre-prepared meals in lightweight sealed packages used as field rations by the military. They can also be used as part of an emergency food supply. The major drawbacks are volume and weight. They can also be a bit on the expensive side (approximately $8 per meal—a one-week supply for two can be purchased for $180–200 if you search for a good deal). All in all, MREs are better items for your Grab-and-Go bag or mobile food supply than a static emergency food pantry. They come completely prepared along with utensils, and can be heated by placing the package in hot water, or by special MRE heaters that you will need to purchase separately.

IA TIP

In 2002, the Feeding Directorate of the Army Soldier Systems Center at Natick, MA developed an improved version of an MRE called the First Strike Ration (FSR). They're specially designed for soldiers in the field that need high levels of energy, nutrition bound together in a lightweight package.

They need no preparation, or even utensils, adding to their ease of use. These aren't yet available for purchase by civilians, but if you're a member of the U.S. military, I would encourage you to add these to your emergency food pantry. Not as the principal content, but a supplement that could be used occasionally.

EFS Storage Area

The area that you choose to set up your emergency food storage area is quite important. It should be in a place that is insect-free, relatively cool and dry (low humidity) with a stable year-round temperature, between 50–72° F and away from direct sunlight to prevent spot heating by sunlight that can accelerate spoilage and break down the storage medium.

It must also be in an area that is safe from flooding. If you live in an earthquake-prone area, anchor your shelves or whatever you use to stack the food on to the walls to prevent it from falling. Temperature is an extremely important dynamic in the area you select for your EFS. For every temperature increase of approximately 20° F, the shelf life of your food is reduced by half. And for each reduction of the temperature by 10° F, you can double the food's shelf life, so this variable should always be factored in when selecting a spot for your food supply.

IA TIP

Large or small food containers can be used if you store your food in an area where there are insects or pests, or which is prone to flooding. Thirty- to 55-gallon plastic storage barrels are great, because your emergency food is protected, and can be moved if necessary. They also keep your food consolidated, and in the worst of times can be sealed and buried if necessary. If you choose this storage method, keep a handcart handy. I prefer keeping my emergency food in barrels, because if needed I can easily move them. Mobility is one of the most important qualities that an EFS can have.

It should also, whenever possible, be kept on shelves and off of the floor, and set with a little air space between the shelf and the wall to maintain air circulation and prevent it from absorbing the heat or cold stored by the surface of the floor or walls, to minimize condensation. This will also help to safeguard it from insects and pests.

IA TIP

Closets work best for small apartments. If you use a closet, find a couple of bricks (of the same size) and a rigid board. Lay the board across the bricks to form a makeshift platform. Place your food on top.

The heaviest food items should be placed at the bottom for easy access—and the lightest at the top. Make labels with a Sharpie marker on masking tape or label-maker, and place them on *every* food item along with the date you placed it there and the projected expiration date of the item.

Your emergency food supply must also be inconspicuous. Visitors, neighbors, and even extended family members should not know that you have one unless you choose to inform them that you do (and I strongly advise against this, unless you are certain that they can keep secrets, and they have their *own* food!)

IA TIP

You will need to create a mobile version of your emergency food supply that can be rapidly moved if a disaster or emergency forces you to evacuate your home. You can use something as simple as a grocery cart and a laundry bag, provided that it is waterproof. Pack the food in levels separated by a section of cardboard or rigid plastic. Depending on the type, size, and number of people you need to feed, each level can contain from one to five days' worth of food. It's a great way to keep the food organized, also.

The laundry bag is also a great disguise. If you're in a situation where you need to use a mobile pantry, you'd better keep it hidden for your own sake. The laundry bag gives you great cover. If you throw in a few pairs of dirty socks and drawers, that'll add to the ruse. The less anyone suspects that you have emergency food, the better.

You might need to cache it away if you need to enter an evacuation center. If you do, find an area with a low amount of human traffic. Place it in the least conspicuous area you can locate. If your food is primarily canned items, you won't have to worry about insects or vermin.

EFS Shelf Life

The shelf life of foods varies dramatically, so choose what you store away wisely. Make sure it's something that you enjoy eating, and which stores well. *Science Daily* has a great article online that I encourage you to read about the shelf life of foods, called "Keeping Food for Years" (www.sciencedaily.com/videos/2007/0208-keeping_food_for_years.htm).

According to the article, scientists at Brigham Young University have determined that "some low-moisture foods such as dried apples can be safe to eat even years after their expiration date, if properly stored." I'd suggest that you conduct some detailed research on the shelf life of various types of food so that you can choose your favorite types, and know exactly when they must be cycled out of emergency food supply.

IA TIP

Like your emergency water supply, your food must also be cycled constantly to guarantee freshness. Start with the first batch in. For every item you eat, replace it with something fresh. This is abbreviated as FIFO—*first in, first out.* If you maintain this practice, you'll always have great-tasting, fresh food.

Since you spent your hard-earned dollars for this book, I'll save you a little time and effort by offering you a list of some commonly used American staple and "comfort" food products that you should include in your emergency food pantry. I realize that the powdered drink mixes are high in sugar and aren't very nutritious (like many of the other products on this list for that matter!), but will come in handy if you were forced to drink purified water for long periods, as it will make it taste a little better. The comfort items are great, because they help you to keep your spirits up during difficult times.

The data is compiled from a combination of info from food storage studies conducted by the University of Illinois, College of Agricultural, Consumer and Environmental Sciences Study, Virginia Tech (see the complete study at www. ext.vt.edu/pubs/foods/348-960/348-960.html), and from my own personal observations.

Comfort Foods (Basic Staple Items).........**With Shelf Life in Months**

- Pasta 24
- Rice (white) 24
- Rice (minute) 18
- Sugar (white) .... Indefinite
- Sugar (brown) 18
- Sugar (confectioners and granulated) .... 24+
- Salt.. Indefinite
- Soup mix 12

- Campbell's soup 12–24
- Pop Tarts... 2-4
- Cornstarch .... 24+
- White flour.. 6–8
- Whole wheat.. 6–8
- Milk (condensed) 12
- Milk (evaporated) 6
- Syrups 12
- Spices (whole) 12
- Spices (ground)... 6
- Canned vegetables.. 24–48
- Nuts (shelled) 4
- Nuts (in shell and packaged).................................. 24
- Canned meats 36
- Canned baby foods 12
- Texturized vegetable protein................................. 12
- Dried vegetables 12
- Salad oils.. 6
- Oil (Crisco or Puritan) 24
- Tea (bags) 36
- Tea (instant) 24
- Corn oil 18
- Shortening ....Indefinite
- Canned tuna, sardines fish and seafood .... 36+
- Mayonnaise 2–3
- Grated parmesan cheese 10
- Molasses, jam, jelly.. 14+
- Marshmallow cream 3–4
- Chocolate.. 12
- Ramen noodles.. 24+
- Vinegar (container with plastic lid) ....Indefinite
- Macaroni and Cheese........................... Expiration date
- Canned fruit juices 6–8
- Mustard 24
- Catsup, chili, and cocktail sauce 18
- Pickles (in jar).. 12–24
- Canned spaghetti sauce .... Expiration date
- Steak sauce 24
- Tabasco sauce... 60
- Cookies (packaged)... 3
- Crackers, pretzels 3

- Jiffy mixes 24
- Grits 12
- Honey 12–24
- Jell-O... 24
- Rice-a-Roni .... Expiration date
- Pasta-Roni .... Expiration date
- Baking powder ....18 or by expiration date
- Stove Top dressing mix....................... Expiration date
- Instant breakfast products....................................... 6
- Pancake mix 6
- Piecrust mix.. 6
- Betty Crocker mixes ....8–12+
- Peanut butter... 6–9
- Popcorn... 24
- Bottled salad dressings...............................10–12
- Baking soda 24
- Bisquick 24
- Chocolate syrup 24
- Cocoa mixes... 8
- Lipton noodles and sauce........................... 12–24
- Cocoa mix 24
- Bouillon (for flavoring)... 24
- Pudding mixes 12
- Casserole mix..9–12
- Powdered eggs (in sealed container)...........Indefinitely
- Herb/spice blends 24
- Bread crumbs and croutons 6
- Biscuit, cornbread, muffin, brownie mixes............ 10
- Coffee (vacuum-packed).. 24
- Cake mixes...6–9
- Canned frosting 3
- Cereals 6–12
- Cereals (ready-to-cook) 6
- Casseroles (complete with ingredients)............10–12
- Powdered drinks 24
- Coca-Cola, Pepsi, carbonated soft drinks (cans).....6–9
- Corn meal 12
- Vinegar 24
- Biscuit, brownie, muffin mix.................................. 9
- Cake mixes... 9
- Pancake mix 6–9

Whatever you choose to use, the quality of food is important. It should only be top-grade, and provide you with high levels of energy and nutrition. Low-quality food is a poor choice due primarily to storage issues. Your emergency food supply will require you to store away unrefrigerated food for relatively long periods (6–12 months). As the food ages, the nutritional content (and taste) diminishes. In some cases, it will degrade to a point where it is practically inedible. Unless, of course, you enjoy eating slimy cardboard.

High-quality food ages better, because the nutritional content doesn't reduce as rapidly (as with the lower-grade type). You'll need as much nutrition as you can get during a crisis, because the high levels of stress will produce a great deal of physical and emotional strain on your body that can be partially offset and controlled by the vitamin content of high-quality food. You should also include essential vitamins (C, B1, B2, B6, B12, D, A, E, and K). I believe high-quality buffered multi-vitamins are best for emergencies. They are easier to digest, and require less space to store.

I also use high-energy food bars in my emergency food supply and my Grab-and-Go bag. My favorites are Nature Valley granola bars and Power Bars. Survival bars are also great—not long on taste, but very high in nutritional content. Datrex (datrex.com) and Mainstay (survivorind.com) make some of the best available. Trail mix is also a great item to have in your supply. (I make my own special trail mix that includes cashews, walnuts, almonds, and granola.)

Nutriment, Ensure, and protein drinks can also be added to your EFS to provide you with the extra energy and nutrition that you may need during periods of high activity and stress.

Your main objective in the creation of an EFS is to make certain that you will have a steady supply of food available if you ever find yourself in a disaster or emergency that disrupts food deliveries for a protracted period.

It takes work, and is a bit of a financial investment, but is worth every dollar and hour you spend putting it together. Get started with yours now!

CHAPTER 9

Urban Gardening

EVERYONE SHOULD ALWAYS HAVE AN ALTERNATE SOURCE OF FOOD OTHER THAN THE LOCAL supermarket or grocery store. After a large-scale disaster, food may not be readily available for long periods. Or, as our global economic meltdown worsens, the prices may become prohibitive, and the quality questionable.

If your living environment permits it, I believe that it is imperative that you should have a vegetable and spice garden that can at the very least provide high-quality produce to supplement your diet. In WWI and II, Americans were encouraged by the government to grow "Victory Gardens" in their backyards. These mini-farms were helpful to the war effort, as they allowed extra produce to be sent to our troops abroad.

According to Revive the Victory Garden (www.victorygarden.org), 20 million Victory Gardens were planted across the nation in 1943, producing nearly one-third of all the vegetables consumed by Americans for the year.

I believe that conditions in our nation merit a rapid revival of this practice for a number of reasons, with the first being that it will allow for greater control over the quality of our food. Many of the vegetables consumed today are genetically modified. These are plants that are altered through the process of genetic engineering to manifest specific traits, such as resistance to temperature variations, disease, herbicides, insects, and many other qualities.

Some of these traits may be desirable, but there are very strong arguments posed by scientists, environmental activists, and federal government officials stating that genetically modified food can in some cases present a number of public health, environmental, and economic hazards that can create many severe consequences for our food supply and society.

I agree with this position, and feel that the rush toward the genetic modification of our food supply is motivated primarily by corporate greed rather than the desire to feed a growing world population.

Whatever side you fall on, a national revival of urban Victory Gardens would eliminate a great deal of this debate by providing people with a readily available and inexpensive source of organically grown food. Even if purchased from local gardeners, organic food is generally less expensive than the type found in supermarkets, because it is grown in your neighborhood and doesn't need to be hauled long distances by fuel-guzzling trucks. Local food production would help reduce global warming.

A growing number of people across the world recognize the importance of urban farming, and have worked very hard to provide us with examples of its potential. Jules Dervaes of Pasadena, CA created an urban homestead on one-fifth of an acre that is so efficient that it yields enough vegetables and fruit to feed a large family, and produce a small surplus. He also created an organization called Path to Freedom (www.pathtofreedom.com) to help promote the self-sufficient lifestyle. The goals are to "educate individuals and families to integrate sustainable living practices and methods into their daily lives."

Will Allen, a former professional basketball player, has an organization named Growing Power, Inc. (www.growingpower.org) that has built a community food center that includes six greenhouses, an aquaponics house, an apiary, and many other functions—all on two acres in Milwaukee, WI. In 2008, Allen was given the prestigious MacArthur Genius Award to help him expand his operation and help other communities set up similar programs.

Patty "The Garden Girl" Moreno has an excellent website (www.gardengirltv.com) that she created to provide the public with information that they can use to help create indoor and outdoor urban gardens and learn many other sustainable living skills. She has several "how-to" videos on the site that can guide individuals through practically every aspect of urban gardening, from setup and composting to planting and harvesting.

Just like *The X-Files* used to say, "the truth is out there,"and with dedicated people like Dervaes, Allen, and Moreno offering their valuable wisdom and information for free, you won't need to look hard to find it. All you need to get started is the will to get it done. To help you along on your journey, this chapter will provide you with the basic details you'll need to set up your project.

First, make a decision about the type of urban garden you plan to create. If you live in a private home that has a lawn, with decent soil, you will be able to get a full-sized vegetable garden together that will produce a significant yield at harvest time.

If you live in an apartment building, co-op, or condo, you obviously can't have a full-sized garden, but you can still have a small urban indoor garden if you are creative and handy. They're easy to get going, and many of the procedures and tools used are the same as an outdoor garden, albeit on a smaller scale.

Once you get comfortable using your newfound skills, you can graduate to a larger outdoor garden. At the end of this chapter, I'll include a list of helpful gardening books. They helped me to hone my green thumb, and I know they'll do the same for you.

Benefits of Indoor Gardening

The indoor environment has a number of advantages over the outdoor. You don't have to worry about insects and pests nearly as much. This minimizes the need for the use of insecticides. Like a greenhouse, your home's environment is closed and temperature controlled.

This provides a more stable environment that will aid the rapid growth of your plants. If your living space has good air circulation and adequate light to aid proper growth (best if you have south-facing windows, or you can add foil or mylar to reflect light), you already have the environment you need to get an indoor garden started.

Indoor Gardening Gear

You'll need some simple tools to help you manage your garden also. The most important items to own are:

- A mini soil cultivator—to help you break up impacted soil in your containers or pots.
- Mini-trowel—to work in the soil along the edges of your plant containers or pots.
- Mini-spade—to dig out the soil.
- Floral snips.
- Pruning shears.
- A mister—to water and keep the plants moist.

You can purchase these items at any local gardening store. If you can't afford to buy them, you can improvise and use a heavy-duty pair of metal scissors or a small pocket knife as floral snips or pruning shears, a large metal serving spoon as a mini-spade, a strong barbeque fork as a soil cultivator, and a fixed-blade knife as a trowel. It won't be the sleekest or best-looking gear, but it will get the job done.

Choice of Plants

Before laying out your little indoor micro-farm, choose the best plants for successful growth within the dynamics of your home. You certainly won't have fields of corn or wheat growing in your living room, but tomatoes, cucumbers and beans are just a few of many types of tasty treats that you can expect to raise and harvest indoors.

The following is a small list of vegetables most appropriate for indoor gardening:

- Leaf lettuce
- Carrots (small rooted)
- Cherry and container tomatoes
- Eggplant
- Spinach
- Baby beets
- Radishes
- Scallions
- Hot peppers, parsley, and other herbs
- Small miracle broccoli
- Mini cabbage
- Sprouts

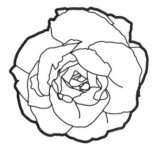

Leaf Lettuce

The Benefits of Sprouts

Of all the indoor vegetables that you can grow, sprouts are the easiest to raise, and the most nutritious. As a living food, their vitamin content actually increases over time, as compared to regular produce that begins to degrade right after it is picked.

Sprouts will continue to grow after being harvested, even while refrigerated. They also produce large amounts of amino acids, enzymes, and minerals. The relative ease and low cost of home sprouting will motivate you to work it to its maximum.

Typically, sprouting seeds cost approximately 25 cents per pound, and can multiply from five to over 14 times their own weight. All you need to get started is a container, some screen, and some seeds, or you can purchase a kit. Wheatgrasskits.com sells an excellent basic and deluxe sprouting kit that comes equipped with everything you need to start your sprout garden.

Purchase Your Seeds

Make certain to use certified organic seeds for your sprouts (and for all your plants). These types are much better to use, because they were grown under strict conditions that dramatically reduce the possibility of contamination from various sources. The certification process isn't perfect, but it is always better to purchase seeds from a company that has some restrictive controls on their production rather than none.

You'll have a much better chance of securing a higher grade of seeds. If you'd like a list of most of the available organic seed varieties, visit the Organic Materials Review Institute's Organic seed database at seeds.omri. org. My own favorite companies are www.mountainroseherbs.com and www. organicseed.com.

"Feed Me, Seymour"—Organic Fertilizer for Your Garden

Other types of vegetable plants have special needs, such as fertilization. Indoor plants don't require as much as outdoor ones, but they still need their regular nitrogen, phosphorous, and potassium meal. Make them happy with some good nutritious organic stuff. For the pre-prepared types, I personally like the product PlanTea (www.plantea.com). This is an odorless organic fertilizer set in little teabags.

IA TIP

During the plants' growth cycle, you'll need to use fertilizer with high nitrogen content.

Once your plants are ready to flower, switch over to a mixture containing higher levels of phosphorous and potassium. They are usually labeled as "bloom" and the levels of chemicals in the mixture are reflected in the ratio numbers on the label. The first number is always smaller than the last two.

You can do more research for other types and brands, but I don't believe you'll find anything easier than this for your first go-round. If you don't mind getting your hands a little dirty, you can even make your own compost by constructing a worm bin. By and large, this is my favorite organic fertilizer.

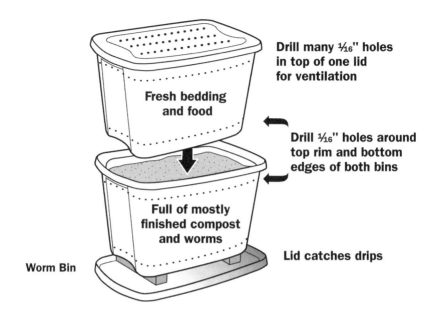

Drill many ¹⁄₁₆" holes in top of one lid for ventilation

Fresh bedding and food

Drill ¹⁄₁₆" holes around top rim and bottom edges of both bins

Full of mostly finished compost and worms

Worm Bin

Lid catches drips

You can purchase an off-the-shelf indoor kitchen composter, but it is so simple and inexpensive to build one from scratch that I don't see the purpose of wasting the extra money that you can use for seeds, tools, or other extras for your little indoor farm. I also believe that it's much better to have a more hands-on approach with your project. It will help build your confidence and experience.

Use the step-by-step process listed here to get your own mini-compost factory started.

Step #1: "Gettin' Wormy Wit It"

Plastic storage bins with sealable lids make excellent "five-star worm hotels." They are cheap and easy to find. The size that you select should be in direct proportion to the amount of kitchen scraps you produce, the amount of plants you will be growing, and the amount of space available in your home. The 2' x 3' x 1' bins work so well for me that I'm going to use them as my template for this project.

Take the lid and either poke or drill twelve 1/4" ventilation holes in the center and repeat this process on the sides of the bin. Make sure that the ventilation holes are uniform and no smaller or larger than 1/4".

Step #2: "Movin' On Up."

Now that you have the hotel rooms ready, you can now collect their occupants. If you live near a yard or large city park, you could go out and forage for worms after a rainstorm, but it would be much easier and quicker if you purchased them from a local gardening store or the Internet. Red worms (*Eisenia fetida* or "wigglers") are best—much better than nightcrawlers, or the Wall Street types. My sources are www.wholesaleworms.com and www.acmewormfarm.com. You need approximately 500 worms (1/2 lb.) for every cubic foot in your bin.

Next step is getting together the bedding material. You can use dried leaves, grass, potting soil, or black and white newspapers (no color because of the dyes, and cut into 1"-wide strips), or an equal combination of them all. You can even use thin cardboard to add a little body to the bedding.

If you want to give your bin a little extra kick, add about a cup of garden soil. You can purchase this at a gardening store, or just find a garden and remove a cup (with the garden owner's permission, of course). The bacteria in the garden soil will help to fire up the worms' digestive systems and help rev up the composting process.

The newspaper, leaves, or cardboard strips will need to be soaked in water until they are damp, then placed at the bottom of the bin. Continue to fill it with the material until it is about 8" deep. Use a spray bottle to keep the bedding material moist if it gets dry as you pack it in.

Step #3: Dinner Is Served.

Once you get your bedding material in the bin, you can begin to collect your kitchen scraps (no leftovers, to avoid odor that can attract flies and other insects) to add in the mix. You can also use unscented and white paper towels, carrot peels, coffee grounds and filters, breads, rice, beans, flowers, and dead plants but never any red meat, poultry, fish, garlic, or foods with oil.

Eggshells are great because they help to maintain proper pH levels in the soil, but they must also be thoroughly rinsed before placing them inside.

Banana peels, apple skins, and fruit are also fantastic worm food, but you will need to wash and scrub them before placing them in the bin. This will get rid of fruit fly eggs and prevent future infestations. Organic bananas and fruit are best because the skins don't contain pesticides. You can even use old tea bags, just as long as you remove the staples. They can injure or kill the worms.

For fruit scraps with a high concentration of water, like melons, you will need to exercise strict controls over the amount you use. This will help to minimize the buildup of odors as they decompose. For the bin size that I suggested earlier, you can use about one to two lbs. of kitchen scraps per week to keep the nutrient supply high and the worms happy.

If your bin is larger, you will need to add more, provided the amount is proportional to the amount of worms and size of bin. Keep in mind that a bin with 2,000 worms (two lbs.) can easily eat through over seven lbs. of kitchen scraps per week.

Store your "vermicuisine" in a sealed plastic bag to prevent odor buildup, or purchase a kitchen compost container. Many models come with an activated charcoal filter to prevent the buildup of odors. Planet Natural (www.planetnatural.com) sells a great model that will help you to collect and store your food without hassles. It will also help to keep the insects away. If they can't smell the food, they can't find it.

At this stage, you are ready to add your worms and cover your kitchen scraps with your selected bedding material. Make sure that you don't leave any food exposed. Use a spray bottle filled with water to keep each layer moist as you lay it out, but be careful not to overdo it and soak the bedding.

Too much moisture can produce odors, and also drown the worms. If the moisture levels get too high, you will need to add more dry bedding to absorb the extra water and restore balance to the mix. You must also be mindful to place the bin in a well-ventilated, quiet, dark area with a temperature that never dips below 50° F or climbs higher than 80° F, and to always keep the contents mixed so that it is properly aerated. The worms can suffocate and die if you don't.

Step #4: Time to Get Growing!

Depending on how much you make, if you use the same size bin that I suggested earlier in the chapter, after about three to six months, the egg shells, banana and orange peels, dried leaves, and vegetables will be converted by the worms into worm castings, technically called vermicompost. It resembles dark soil. Once it reaches this stage, you must harvest (remove) it.

If you own a tarp, old vinyl tablecloth, or any other washable non-porous surface, dump the compost out onto it. You can even use old newspaper. Scoop out equal amounts of compost from the large pile and separate it into smaller sections. Make sure that the room is well lit. This will help you to see the worms and motivate them to move so that you can collect them easier.

Brush away the edges on each small section until the worms begin moving toward the center. Carefully grab the worms and place them back inside the bin, along with extra new bedding to replace the portions removed. Scoop up the brushed-away vermicompost and place it in a container with a lid. Make sure that there aren't any worms left before you close it up!

Your worm bin is also really easy to maintain. When you remove your vermicompost, push it to one side of the bin and add the new bedding material on the other side along with the kitchen scraps. The worms will migrate to the other side in search of the new food. Depending on the size of your bin, you can do this from two to four times per year.

Take the vermicompost and use it as a thin top layer in your potted plants. Sprinkle little bits of it on your seedbeds, and dilute about two tablespoons in one liter of non-chlorinated water to create your own organic fertilizer spray. It's mild enough so that it won't fry your roots. Now that you know the rules, you're ready to make and use top-notch organic fertilizer the way Mother Nature intended!

A Dirty Plant Is an Unhappy Plant

Besides feeding them, you must keep your indoor plants clean. The same dust you find settling on your computer screen will also collect on your plants, inhibiting their growth. Fill a spray bottle with non-chlorinated water, set it on mist, and spray it on your plants. Then take a clean rag and gently wipe the dust away.

That's all it takes to keep them clean and growing fast, the organic no-contaminants way.

Plant Containers

The container that you select is also very important. You must choose a size that conforms to the type of plant that you are growing. Make certain to choose a pot that is large enough to accommodate the plant roots and soil comfortably. If it is too big or small, the plant will grow incorrectly. It must also have drainage holes (approximately 1/2" in diameter) and wide openings. When the container is filled with your plant and soil, make certain to use old newspaper or a chemical-free rag or fabric to prevent the loss of your potting soil.

Clay pots are great, but they require frequent watering because they are porous and tend to absorb water. Plastic or metal containers are better because they retain the water, although UV radiation from the sun can tend to degrade the plastic over time. I personally prefer metal over plastic, but you should use whatever works best for you.

You can improvise, save money, and help the environment by using old coffee cans for small plants and spices and larger cans for the bigger plants. I use old, discarded three-liter olive oil cans, thoroughly wash them out, cut a quarter of the can top off, cut drainage holes in the bottom, carefully fold down the sharp edges while wearing work gloves to avoid injury, and then fill them with soil. These are great for apartments because you can arrange them side-by-side, or even place them in corners to make the best use of your space.

For more info about plant containers, go to www.gardenguides.com.

Plant Stands

You can also place your pots in movable stands with wheels. This is great if you need to move them away from windows, or move them closer to a light source. They come in many different sizes, ranging from small to large, and some have grow lights built into them. The best are constructed with aluminum metal tubing, have wheels and can be fitted with grow lights if necessary. Plant stands can be purchased at gardening stores, or can even be purchased online. Indoorgardensupplies.com has a wide selection of plant stands.

Let There Be Light

Outside of watering your plants, providing them with the proper type of light will be one of your most important tasks as you set up your garden. You have one of two choices: either set it up near windows where the plants can be exposed to the sun, or purchase special "grow" lights that will give them essentially the same type of "full spectrum" light the sun produces… except for the fact that you're paying for it.

Among the best and most energy-efficient lights are compact fluorescent lightbulbs (CFLs). They consume much less energy than their standard counterparts (metal halide, high-pressure sodium/HPS lights), take up less space, and can last for up to 10,000 hours. They also work well with solar and other alternative energy power systems, because they don't consume as much power as other types of grow lights.

LED Grow Lights are even more energy-efficient than CFLs. GlowPanel has a model that is extremely energy-efficient and emits very little heat. They last for up to 50,000 hours and come with a hanging kit that will get you ready to "glow." They're available at www.herbkits.com.

Your garden will need between six to eight hours of daily light to promote proper growth. The amount varies from plant to plant, but for the most part you must stick to the six-to-eight-hour rule to insure that they are getting the appropriate amount. During the winter months, if you situate your garden near a window, you must be very careful to make sure that there are no drafts. If your windows are large and not insulated, cold can radiate from the surface and harm the plants.

You can remedy this by sealing all the drafty cracks and holes, or use grow lights exclusively during the winter months. Not only will they provide the light the plants need, but also a bit of extra heat. You must also make sure that your window garden can be quickly moved aside if you ever experience an emergency where you need to make a rapid exit.

Light requirements for indoor vegetable growing:

- Beans—8 hours light
- Carrots—6 hour minimum
- Beets—6–8 hour minimum
- Cabbage—6 hours
- Kale—6 hours
- Leaf lettuce—6 hours
- Eggplant—8 hours
- Cucumbers—8 hours
- Onions—6 hours
- Peppers—8 hours
- Radishes—6 hours
- Squash—8 hours
- Tomatoes—8 hours
- Turnips—6 hours

Indoor Garden Soil Tips

The soil you use for an indoor garden is also very important. Regular garden soil isn't recommended. It may be laden with insects and their larvae, toxins, diseases, debris particles, and other undesirable contaminants. This is especially true if the soil you choose is collected from someplace near, or inside of a garden in a large city.

It also doesn't pack well into containers, and has a tendency to compact over time. Your best bet for indoor garden soil would be a mixture of equal parts peat, perlite, vermiculite, and potting soil. The pH level of the soil can be adjusted by adding one teaspoon of hydrated lime for every gallon of soil that is mixed together.

Your indoor garden may still attract certain insect pests that are attracted to houseplants. Always have some organic insecticidal soap on hand to help keep them clean. You can also use diatomaceous earth (a stabilizing ingredient in dynamite!). I find it quite amusing that it can also be used to "bomb" out insects from your garden. A light dusting over your plants will keep most pests away.

It's organic and non-toxic, so you don't have to be concerned about children or pets that may come in contact with it. The plants will need to be watered every day. You can get away with skipping days, but *not* during the winter months, when your windows are closed and your apartment is heated.

This sucks away humidity and can have a tendency to dehydrate your plants. You must also make certain to maintain balance with the plant nutrients, because the extra watering tends to flush away the fertilizer.

Plant Pollination

Plants that have a male and female flower will need to be pollinated. This can be achieved by taking a small fiber paint/make-up brush, or Q-tip, and literally hand-transferring pollen from male plants to female (male plants have stamens, the pollen-producing reproductive organ, and females have pistils, the seed-producing part of a flower).

You must remember that each time you switch the plant type that you're pollinating, you've got to thoroughly clean off your brushes. Some plants, such as tomatoes, will only need to be shaken every two or three days to simulate pollination. Others, like beans and peas, self-pollinate. If you have serious plant allergies, it wouldn't be wise to grow these types of plants in your indoor garden unless you place an air filter or ionizer near your grow space.

Balancing Your Environment

Plants need different conditions to grow in. Some, like leaf crops, thrive in cooler temperatures. Others, such as tomatoes, need warmer environments with more light. You will need to decide on the type of plant that is best suited for the conditions in your home. Make an assessment of your living environment, e.g., the average temperature for the length of the grow season you choose, moisture content or "dew point," and available light.

You might want to add oscillating fans to aid in air circulation. This helps a process called transpiration (the evaporation of water from plant surfaces), and it also helps to strengthen the plants.

If you choose multiple types of plants that require different growing conditions, select specific areas where the temperature and light can be altered and controlled to accommodate them. If you don't mind the extra labor, you can build small terrarium-style enclosures that will allow you to create "micro-climates."

This will allow you to adjust the temperature and moisture content to suit the particular plant's growing needs. Purchase some transparent plastic sheets at your local hardware store. Measure the area around the pots or stands, and cut them to the matching dimensions. Build some light wooden or wire framing that conforms around your pots or containers, and drape the plastic over it when completed.

Hydroponics

If you want to get even more technical, you could move into another indoor growing method called hydroponics. This technique allows you to grow your plants without any soil. The plants draw from a nutrient-rich solution of water and sand, gravel, or any material that can easily retain and allow for drainage of water.

It might seem like something out of a sci-fi film, but, hydroponics have been around for millennia. There are Egyptian hieroglyphic records of priests growing plants in water. The Aztecs had "floating gardens," and the ancient Babylonians had "hanging gardens" that all utilized hydroponic growing techniques.

Hydroponic systems have a number of distinct advantages over regular indoor growing methods, but require more attention to the details. Because they don't use soil, they're not vulnerable to pests. Hydroponic gardens don't produce odors. The plants can be grown very close together, or can be rigged to hang from walls, ceilings, or anything that your imagination and gravity will allow. They also grow much faster.

Hydroponic gardens have a much stricter standard regarding nutrients, light, and even the air flowing between the roots. Because they are exposed to more air than when they are buried in regular soil, you must be very cautious to prevent them from dehydrating. If this happens, the plants will no longer have the ability to draw water and nutrients. This will cause them to rapidly dry up and die.

To start a hydroponic garden, you can use any type of pot or container that is watertight. It can be homemade or manufactured. You will also need grow lights to help maintain a steady supply of light, and a growing medium, i.e., something that your plant can grow in. There are many different types of natural and even human-made growing mediums.

Even plain old air can work if you set up your system correctly. The type you choose is largely dependent on what you plan to grow, the type of system you are working with (homemade or manufactured), your home environment, and other conditions. The most frequently used growing mediums are listed below:

- Air
- Sand
- L.E.C.A. (Light Expanded Clay Aggregate)
- Sawdust
- Fiberglass insulation
- Water
- Gravel
- Rockwool
- Perlite—One of the best hydroponic growth mediums available. Usually mixed together with vermiculite in a 50/50 ratio. Biggest drawback is that it doesn't hold water well, so it dries rapidly, and the dust can be irritating—especially for people with respiratory problems.
- Lava rock
- Oasis cubes—These are small cubes that are specifically designed to promote vegetative propagation, great for when you grow straight from seed or cuttings.
- Vermiculite—No relation to vermicompost; this is a natural mineral that expands with heat.
- Coconut Fiber—The organic waste product of the coconut industry is one of the most popular growing mediums. It has many properties that help to stimulate plant growth. It has hormones that stimulate roots and protection against fungus infestation and other diseases. When used in a 50/50 mixture with expanded clay pellets, it is considered by many to be the perfect growth medium. When purchasing coconut fiber, always make sure to stick with the highest grade. Less expensive types contain fiber impregnated with sea salt and other preserving agents that reduce its effectiveness as a growth agent.
- Sphagnum Moss

Your hydroponic garden can either be *active* or *passive*. Active hydroponic gardens use electric pumps to circulate nutrients. There are a number of different types, including top feed, aeroponics, sub-aeration, nutrient film technique, and ebb and flow.

Passive gardens use different nutrient transference mechanisms such as absorbent materials or even hydroponic absorption wicks (found at most garden stores). They use capillary action (liquid moving upward against gravitational force) to deliver the nutrients to the plants.

Since the active types depend on electricity, you must consider the fact that during power failures, you will need to manually circulate the nutrients, or, if you have a renewable energy system (solar panels, wind, etc.) you must calculate the amount of energy consumed by the pumps and factor that into the design of your system. For beginners, I recommend passive hydroponic systems.

Passive Planter Hydroponic Garden Set-Up

You'll need a one-gallon clean planting pot or container that has drainage holes, or you will need to add them yourself with a drill, scissor, or other sharp object (make sure to wear work gloves when making holes to avoid cutting your hands). You'll also need a bucket (one gallon) to serve as a reservoir for the nutrients.

Fill the container with a growth medium (up to 2" from the rim) such as the types described earlier in this section. Take your plant and place it in the container in the same way you would if you were using soil.

In your next step, you'll need the bucket to function as the base. Fill this with the nutrient solution pre-balanced with the proper pH level for the plants. Set the pot or plant container right into the nutrient solution.

You can also use a hydroponic wick system to deliver the nutrients to the roots of the plants. Take your hydroponic growing wick and place it inside the pot or container. Line the walls as you insert it, making sure that it passes through the drainage holes, hanging on the outside.

The wick length must be long enough to extend to the reservoir. The container or pot will be placed between 5–8" above it to allow for the capillary action to work properly and draw the nutrients into the plants.

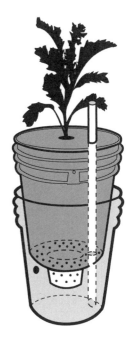

Passive Hydroponic Planter

The next step will be filling the plant containers with your medium of choice to the same levels (2" from the top) as mentioned earlier. You'll also need to purchase, or even construct, a table with a hole in the center that is large enough for you to place your container over the nutrient reservoir and slip the wick through it.

Once you slide it through the hole, put the reservoir under the table, directly beneath your container. Take the wick and place it in the reservoir. Watch and feel the wick to make sure that it is absorbing the water properly.

Make sure that the reservoir is filled to about 1 1/2" from the top. After about one hour, place your hand inside your container to check and see if the medium is moist. Once it is, you are ready to add the nutrient mixture, and begin to grow your vegetables.

The plants you choose for your hydroponic grow system are very important. You should select species that grow well together and have similar environmental considerations, such as temperature, light, and the nutrient mix.

The advantages of a passive hydroponic system are:

- They don't require mechanical equipment and electrical power. An average sized system takes about eight minutes a day to make sure that the nutrient and pH levels are correct.
- They are extremely inexpensive.
- Very easy to set up and maintain.

However, the disadvantages are:

- Active systems have a higher growth rate.
- Not as efficient as active systems.
- The reservoirs must be changed about every two weeks and replaced with new nutrients.
- Since plants grown in *all* hydroponic kits have smaller root systems, certain plants such as tomatoes and other fruiting plants will need extra support that you will need to create.
- The grow lights will raise your electrical bill, or add to the load of your renewable energy system.

All in all, if you are ready to put in a little extra time and work, hydroponic gardens are a fantastic alternative to the traditional indoor gardening methods. If you get really good at it, you'll be quite surprised by the number of high quality organic vegetables and other plants you can grow indoors.

Specialty Indoor Vegetable Growing Kit Products

There are also a number of consumer products available that help you to grow vegetables indoors. Some of them even pop up on late night TV infomercials. The best that I have ever seen, and am quite familiar with, is the AeroGarden (www.aerogrow.com and www.aerogardenstore.com). This is a fully automated mini hydroponicum (hydroponic growing box) that you can use to grow herbs, and many other types of vegetables. It's easy to use, because a computer chip controls every process of the growing cycle.

The grow lights are built in, and it's small enough to place on a tabletop. It's a great product that you can use to complement your indoor garden, but should not be used as a replacement for your full-sized project. This is because it does not provide you with a medium to learn and practice your indoor gardening skills, because *everything* is automatic.

It does help to illustrate just how easy it is to grow food indoors, and can motivate you to build a much larger indoor garden.

I mentioned at the beginning of the chapter that I would include a number of books that I have used to help me develop my indoor and outdoor gardening skills.

Indoor Gardening:

- *Four-Season Harvest: Organic Vegetables from Your Home Garden All Year Long*, Eliot Coleman and Barbara Damrosch.
- *The Insatiable Gardener's Guide: How to Grow Anything and Everything Indoors, Year Round,* Susan Brackney.
- *Gardening Indoors; Gardening Indoors with Soil and Hydroponics; Hydroponic Basics,* George Van Patten.
- *Urban Eden: Grow Delicious Fruit, Vegetables and Herbs in a Really Small Space,* Adam and James Caplin.

Outdoor Gardening:

- *Square Foot Gardening*, Mel Bartholomew.
- *The Gardener's A-Z Guide to Growing Organic Food*, Tanya L.K. Denckla.
- *The New Organic Grower,* Eliot Coleman.
- *Organic Gardening for Dummies,* Ann Whitman.
- *Gardening Basics for Dummies,* Steven A. Frowine.

CHAPTER 10

Shelter

NEXT TO WATER, SHELTER IS THE MOST IMPORTANT SURVIVAL NECESSITY. FOOD COMES LAST on the list of essentials because you can survive for weeks without it. For long- and short-term survival situations, especially in harsh environments, shelter is a more urgent need. During emergencies or mass evacuations, you may find yourself spending time outdoors, exposed to the elements and anything else that may be in the air (fallout, toxic smoke, disease-carrying mosquitoes). You will need portable shelter, or the know-how to find or construct shelter.

Tents

A good tent will provide sufficient protection until you find more permanent shelter. Many types of tents are available, including camping, hunting, military, and expedition tents, even geodesic domes. Not only does a tent provide pro- tection from the elements, it can also give you a little privacy in a crowded Red Cross evacuation center or outdoor area.

Tents for emergency shelter during evacuation should have the following characteristics:

- Low weight.
- Durability. A flimsy tent that flies apart in a strong wind or a rainstorm is useless.
- Ease and speed of set-up.
- A size that suits your needs. A crowded tent increases wear and tear on the material; one too large wastes space and weight.
- Flame-retardant material. It should meet C.P.A.I.-84 specifications and be coated with flame-retardant spray.
- Cost. Look for a deal, but don't give up any of the aforementioned features.

Makers of high-quality tents include Coleman, North Face, Eureka, Kelty, Apache Instant Tents (sets up in one minute), and Cabela's.

If a regular camping tent isn't enough for you, a geodesic expedition dome tent is the next best thing to a permanent structure. Geodesic dome tents are strong and can remain standing in winds over 50 mph. The only drawbacks are weight (portability) and price (about $500). If you have deep pockets, you can purchase the North Face 2-Meter Dome. It sleeps eight, can withstand 70 mph wind and costs a steep $5,000. Companies such as Shelter Systems (www.shelter-systems.com) offer even larger geodesic-type structures for emergency shelter.

Domes

At Burning Man in the Nevada Black Rock desert, dozens of festivalgoers construct 20' geodesic dome shelters out of conduit pipe. These are by far the most stable emergency structures. When firmly anchored, they can easily withstand desert winds in excess of 70 mph. If you are handy with tools, this type of emergency shelter are inexpensive and relatively simple to construct. If your home is leveled by an earthquake or hurricane, a dome like this will keep you and even a large family sheltered for months, if necessary.

A 24' dome with a nearly 9' ceiling constructed from ¾" conduit pipe (available at hardware stores for approximately $3 per 10' section), costs a total of about $350 provided you already have power tools and a vise to flatten conduit pipe ends. For cutting pipe a Milwaukee Sawzall or circular saw fitted with a metal cutting disc works best. Once completed, the Geodesic Dome weighs 300 lbs., light enough for two strong people to carry disassembled.

With the right tools and help, this geodesic structure can be built and covered with tarp in two days or less (depending on your level of experience with tools). I completed my first dome in slightly less than 18 hours. My son built his first dome constructed from newspaper when he was six years old, proving to those who watched him that emergency geodesic dome shelters can be built by anyone.

Geodomes are the perfect temporary (or permanent) structures. They should be built before disasters strike and stored away for use if needed.

www.desertdomes.com, a site by Tara Landry, a mechanical engineer and Burning Man domebuilder, provides useful information about how to build electrical conduit domes, their cost and links to other helpful dome building sites.

If you prefer to buy a pre-manufactured emergency shelter, Pacific Domes (www.pacificdomes.com) offer some of the best reasonably-priced domes ranging from 16' to 60' diameters. All come complete with a galvanized steel frame, fabric cover and doors.

Another less expensive emergency shelter called a Hexayurt combines geodesic principles and a yurt, the traditional homes of Mongolian nomads. Hexayurts can be built in less than one day. Visit www.mindismoving.org/hexayurt to learn more.

www.thepod.net offers prefabricated "Hexayurt and Geodome" type modular structures called Icopods and Decapods. They were invented by Sanford Ponder, a visionary artist who wanted to create a low cost and easy-to-construct method of building emergency shelter. Ponder also created Icosa Village (www.icosavillage.com) to help distribute the pods to relief organizations.

If One Becomes Homeless

As we witnessed in New Orleans, our government is not prepared to deal with the displacement of a large number of people. Hurricane Katrina was an awful event, but other natural and unnatural catastrophes could force far greater numbers to become homeless wanderers in desperate search of decent shelter.

A terrorist strike against the Indian Point nuclear facility near New York City could provoke a forced mass evacuation of nearly 12 million. Al Qaeda operatives have been arrested with detailed information on nuclear plants.

The second richest man in the free world, Warren Buffett, media tycoon Ted Turner, and former senator Sam Nunn have teamed up to create the Nuclear Threat Initiative (www.nti.org) in hopes that they can influence the government to take this threat seriously. If we can barely handle one million hurricane evacuees under controlled conditions, what would we do with three, five or ten million? Our government would be overwhelmed and forced to activate harsh continuity of government (COG) laws that would convert our country into an actual police state.

The economic repercussions of this type of mega-disaster would be severe, putting millions of people out of work and leaving them destitute. Many would be forced onto the streets, fighting to survive any way that they could.

This is why you must learn, at the very least, the basic protocols on securing emergency shelter if you ever become homeless.

Should you ever search for temporary shelter you will find that most urban shelters are overcrowded, unsafe and filthy. Private shelters and churches are better managed, but most will be filled to the limit. If you don't have friends or family to stay with if you find yourself homeless, use your time to:

- Check your local homeless assistance programs. Every city has some kind of program. Find one that immediately offers food and shelter, especially if you have a family.
- Apply for transitional housing and Section 8. The applications take time to process, and the recent real estate bubble has many landlords refusing Section 8 applications, but the sooner you apply, the greater your chances of eventually obtaining an apartment with affordable rent.
- Set up a post office box for mail delivery. You will need a method of picking up your mail. Friends and family will be able to keep in touch while you are struggling to build back your life.
- Use your public library to maintain an e-mail account. This provides you with another method of maintaining contact with friends, family, and potential employers.
- Make sure that you secure ID if you lost it. You will need ID to enter most shelters.
- Try to find a safe place to store your Grab-and-Go Bags. Friends and acquaintances may not be able to let you stay in their homes, but will let you leave your important personal items (Grab-and-Go Bag, important papers, etc.). If you can't find a place for your stuff, locate an inexpensive storage facility and leave your critical items there until you can find a safe place to stay.

Make a prompt decision when a temporary shelter alternative becomes available. The conditions of most temporary shelters I have seen in New York City are miserable, but the environment on the streets is in most cases far worse. Camping out on the streets, subway tunnel, railroad yard, highway underpass, empty lot, or even inside an abandoned building is a dangerous choice. If you are forced by circumstance to sleep outside, choose a location with frequent pedestrian traffic—the more, the better. You have probably heard about the nasty things that happen to homeless people in deserted areas of our cities.

If you seek temporary shelter in an abandoned building, make a thorough investigation of the structure in the daytime and make sure that it is empty and relatively intact. Take note of holes, shaky staircases, protruding sharp objects, and other hazards that could be tripped over, bumped into, or fallen on once it is dark. Remove any garbage and waste material from the area you will use, and find another location in the building for your bodily wastes and garbage.

Block off the front door and other points of entry before you sign off for the night. Leave something near a door or window that would be knocked down by someone trying to pass through the area while you are asleep. This is a low-tech alarm. Violent encounters are possible if you use abandoned buildings for shelter. Remember, abandoned buildings are like rest stops for drug addicts, the mentally disturbed and other potential assailants.

You must also remember that when you take shelter in an abandoned building, you are living on someone else's property illegally and can be arrested for trespassing. There are some squatting laws that vary from city to city and state to state. A few provide you with some rights but you will need to investigate what they are.

The recent string of disasters around the world has shown all of us the importance of having very comprehensive personal emergency shelter plans in place. Do not wait for the next disaster to strike before you get yours together.

CHAPTER 11

Sanitation and Hygiene

"Toilet out of order, please use floor below."

—Anonymous

ONE OF THE FIRST PROBLEMS ENCOUNTERED DURING DISASTERS OCCURS THE FIRST TIME YOU need to use a bathroom and there aren't any available. Then you'll be forced to find an area where you can comfortably (or not so comfortably) answer nature's call and clean yourself up afterward. This will be particularly difficult if you are on the run or stuck somewhere like the Katrina evacuees who were forced to live inside the world's biggest public toilets—otherwise known as the New Orleans Convention Center and Superdome.

Even if you can find a decent space to take care of business, you probably won't have access to toilet paper or a sink. This is when personal hygiene begins to suffer and, depending on the severity of the emergency, will rapidly degenerate. Worse still, you might be forced to live with thousands of others in the same condition. Eventually, these unhygienic conditions will cause illnesses and disease, especially with people who have compromised immune systems, the elderly and children. Do you need more reasons why you must develop your own emergency sanitation plan?

Any major disaster will disrupt water distribution. Even if some water remains available, it will probably be needed for drinking and cooking. When you cannot use a flush toilet, you must have a system in place that will allow you to deal with the short-term and long-term waster disposal situations.

The best way to begin your emergency sanitation program is to recognize the importance of carrying personal hygiene items in your Grab-and-Go Bag that will allow you to keep clean for a at least 72 hours. Please refer to Chapters 3 and 4 for details on sanitation and hygiene items you should include in your E-Kit and Grab-and-Go Bag. The products listed below are recommended for inclusion in your Grab-and-Go Bag.

- Travel packages of moist towelettes and hand sanitizers. I carry the moist towelettes called Hoo-Ahhs and ReadyBath. Hoo-Ahhs were specially developed by the military for field soldiers. They are tougher than most other wipes and can be used to keep your entire body clean. ReadyBath are pre-moistened washcloths that can be heated by microwave heaters, the sun or Flameless Ration Heaters (used primarily by the military or by campers to heat MRE servings). Hoo-Ahhs have 20 large 7"× 10" wipes per pack. ReadyBath has eight—two packs should be more than enough to get you through a three day period. These are a bit too large to carry in your E-Kit but are great to include in your Grab-and-Go Bag. I also like to carry a small bottle of Dr. Bronner's Peppermint soap. You can lather up with a small amount of water and it easily rinses away. (If you are allergic to coconut oil, do not buy this product.) If you have long hair, you might also want to purchase a product called ReadyBath Shampoo and Conditioning Cap. This is a disposable one-time use cap that you can use to wash your hair.

IA TIP

If toilet paper or moist towelettes are not available, but clean water is, you can improvise a spray bottle that you can use to clean yourself up that actually works better than toilet paper. Find a half-liter or liter water bottle. Remove its cap and use the hole-puncher in your multi-tool to make six holes in a tight circular pattern. Add water, and screw the cap on tightly. If you squeeze hard, you will produce a strong stream of water that can effectively clean off your hindquarters with no trouble. Sports-cap bottles work to similar effect.

- Ziploc 1-quart storage bags are also great items to carry. In a pinch, they can be used as small urinals that will allow you to discreetly answer nature's call. Ziploc bags can hold upwards of 20 oz. of liquid. They can also be sealed up and thrown away. Larger plastic bags can be used to store solid waste.
- Don't forget to include chlorophyll tablets in your emergency sanitation supply bag. They can dramatically reduce fecal odor. This can be a crucial item to have if you are in a situation where raw human wastes cannot be disposed of properly, or if you care for an elderly or sick family member. You simply swallow them and they work their magic in your GI tract.

All of these items can be easily carried in small pocket-sized pouches. My own toiletries kit contains all of the listed materials and a few extras including some aromatherapy oils, mints, and toothpicks.

Staying clean during a disaster is a matter of physical and psychological health. Losing your ability to maintain proper hygiene can make a bad situation worse. Keeping these items handy is a minor inconvenience. But if you ever find yourself in a situation where you need them, you will find out how quickly that inconvenience becomes a blessing.

For prolonged emergencies that extend beyond one week, you will need to learn methods of human waste disposal. If you are living in a home or apartment, chemical waste treatment is best.

Chemical Waste Treatment Methods

To treat and dispose of human waste with chemicals, you will need:

- One five gallon bucket; if you have a large family, you will need more.
- Chlorine bleach (Clorox is best), industrial-strength disinfectant, liquid detergent.
- Moist towelettes, toilet paper.
- Heavy-duty plastic garbage bags and ties.

If you are in an area with a usable toilet bowl that isn't backed up, you can put a garbage bag inside the bowl, using it as lining. Otherwise, use the bag to line a bucket. If you can, find an old toilet seat, or four boards nailed together to form a square that fits over the top of the bucket. Add a 2' × 2' square piece of wood with a hole cut in the center. After using, pour disinfectant into the spoiled bag. Remove the bag from the bucket or toilet, and seal it tightly. Find a safe, cool, insect-free waste disposal area free of all sharp objects, food, moisture, and cats and dogs (pets can smell the contents and tear the bags open).

The best disinfectant to neutralize harmful bacteria found in stool is chlorine bleach. You should pre-prepare a special solution of one part liquid chlorine bleach to ten parts water. If you have more than a dozen people using this waste disposal method, I suggest keeping a supply of the powerful germicidal agent called Encore handy. This is an EPA-registered disinfectant, virucide, cleaner, mildewstat and deodorizer. It destroys HIV-1, athlete's foot fungus and many other bacteria.

More effective disinfectants: HTH (high-test calcium hypochlorite), available at most swimming pool supply stores; powdered chlorinated lime, which is available at building supply stores; and, of course, the old standard, Lysol.

Kitty litter can also be used to stabilize the waste. Odor and moisture absorbing Tidy Cat works quite well. Just drop a large heaping scoop into the bag before and after use. Follow the same process described earlier to dispose of the waste.

Once you stabilize the waste, you need to get rid of it. You can begin by digging a pit that is a minimum of 100 feet from any well, water pipes, spring, food storage or living area. It must be three to four feet deep, and if possible, on the downhill side of your home or shelter. If you are lucky enough to find an old 55-gallon drum, you can pour the wastes inside of it (wear your R-100 respirator, gloves and protective clothing). Bury the drum to prevent the leaching of the waste into the surrounding soil. Line the pit with newspapers to absorb some of the liquid.

If a lid for the 55-gallon drum cannot be found, use a trash bag. Draw it tightly across the top of the drum like a membrane and use duct tape to seal it tightly. If no barrels can be found, puncture a hole into a bag of waste to release air and drop it in the pit. Line the pit with newspapers first—they will absorb some of the liquid, preventing it from leaching into the surrounding soil.

Porta-Potties

We are all familiar with the "porta-potties" that we see at sporting events and rock concerts. They are also used when disasters break down our water distribution and filtration systems. These toilets use strong chemical solutions to eliminate odor and disinfect the waste material. There are a number of smaller units for the home that work in the same way. The downside is that the waste material is full of dangerous chemicals such as formaldehyde, and they can be difficult to dispose.

Biological Waste Treatment Methods

Biological waste treatment is when organisms break down the waste, converting it into compost. This is my preferred method of waste disposal because it does not harm the environment.

Stool Digesters

Many different products use enzyme mixes and bacteria for waste management. Many can even be used in portable/emergency toilets and waste disposal pits. Organic digesters accelerate the decomposition of human waste into fertilizer. Here are a few:

- Earth's Balance "Dogonit" Stool Destroyer
- Lim'nate Stool Liquefier
- Doggie Dooley Stool Liquefier

The products above are designed to treat dog waste in small septic tanks. Once the waste is placed into the tank, the bacterial cultures and enzymes liquefy the stool, then leach it into the ground harmlessly. If you live in an area that allows this type of waste disposal, I suggest you purchase a dog stool digester and have it on standby. They are surprisingly affordable.

If You Choose to Use a Biological Method of Waste Disposal:

- Do not use chlorinated water to dilute the stool; this will kill necessary bacteria in the digester.
- Test the soil in your area. If it is mostly clay, you will have poor drainage and this can interfere with the digestive process. To test your soil, dig a hole approximately 2' × 2' about one foot deep. Pour a bucket of water inside. This should take about two days to drain. If it does, your system is in the clear. If it doesn't, you won't be able to use this method.
- The hotter the climate, the better this method will work. If you live in a cold climate, or it is winter, you will need to use chemical waste disposal methods.

Improvised Stool Digester

If you don't want to go the route of purchasing a mini septic tank, a large bucket (preferably metal) can be used. All you need to do is poke about 100 small holes in a ring of about five concentric circles at the bottom of the bucket and sink it into the ground. Place the stool and digester inside and close the lid tightly. If you don't overload it, it will get the job done almost as well as the mini septic tank.

Latrines

A latrine is used when a larger number of people need an effective method of human waste management. It is a non-chemical option. The simplest form is called a "cathole." To build one, dig a hole about 6" deep and 1' wide. Waste should be dropped in this hole, and covered with earth. The microorganisms in the topsoil are used to break down the waste material. It will decompose in about three days to a week. Catholes are too small to be used by more than six people for more than two days.

The more people use the same cathole, its circle needs to be dug wider, not deeper. The organisms that decompose the waste are only found in topsoil. If you decide to use a cathole, make sure that it is at a minimum 200' from water, your base camp, food storage area, or water source.

If you need something larger to support more people for a longer period of time, you will need to build a large trench or pit latrine.

Trench Latrine

Trench latrines are designed specifically to be temporary waste disposal methods for emergencies. They are quick and easy to build and simple to use. But, because of their open-air nature, they are only desirable if no other alternative waste disposal methods are available.

To Build a Trench Latrine, You Will Need:

- Wood panels, tin, or plastic sheeting for fence.
- Water container with tap and soap.
- Drainage stones.
- Staggered entrance.

- Planks.
- Trenches (width: 3', depth: 3½–4').
- Soil for the burial of human waste.
- Shovels, hammers, picks, duct tape, baling wire (for fence posts).
- Planks (or wooden poles).
- Stakes (for the fence).
- Plastic sheeting (or local material).
- Empty cans (to handle soil for burying excreta).
- Water container (*e.g.,* 200-liter drum) with tap.
- Soap.

Installation:

- Build at least 250' away from water storage areas and downhill from them.
- Dig the trenches about 3' wide and 4' deep. Allow about 40" per 100 users. Leave a good amount of excavated soil at the side of each trench so users can cover their waste with it after each use. This will reduce the numbers of insects and flies drawn to the area by the odor of the excreta.

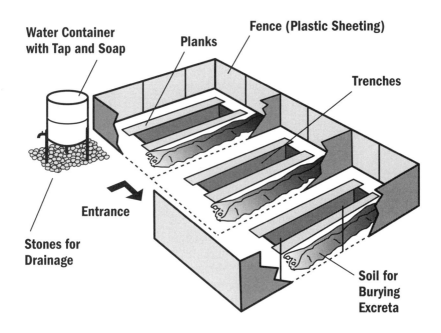

Water Container with Tap and Soap

Planks

Fence (Plastic Sheeting)

Trenches

Entrance

Stones for Drainage

Soil for Burying Excreta

- Lay wooden planks along the two sides to guarantee a good foothold. This will also limit the erosion of the trench edges. When the waste reaches about 3' from the surface, fill in the trench with earth and compact it with the back of a shovel. When finished, you must mark the area and dig another trench.
- Place a fence around the area (posts or planks with plastic sheeting such as shower curtains attached), and put up a staggered entrance-way to cut down on the risk of animals straying inside. This will also help to maintain some level of privacy for the users.
- Place a water container along with soap in a visible spot to encourage use.

Important

- Make sure that your shelter or base camp is not downwind of the trench area.
- Wooden poles can be used in place of wooden planks. If used, they must be buried approximately eight to ten inches.
- Build separate areas for males and females.

Homemade Composting Toilet

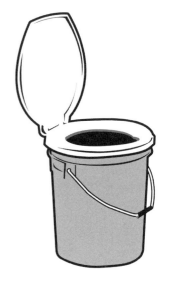

This waste disposal and recycling method is only suited for the worst case scenario type of disaster. The most practical human waste composting system would be a "sawdust toilet." The great thing about this method is that it is chemical-free, only requires sawdust, and converts human feces and urine into something that is reusable as fertilizer. The problem is that it produces strong odors when you are getting it started. If you use it, make sure that you do it properly and in a well-ventilated area.

To begin, your feces and urine must be collected in a bucket with a lid. After every use, cover the waste with sawdust, dried leaves, peat moss or very dry soil. Once the bucket is filled, the contents must be transferred to a compost bin (available at most gardening supply stores). This should be a bottomless two-chambered model.

The covering material helps to reduce the odors and also to supply the carbon needed by the organisms to decompose the waste and balance the nitrogen levels of the urine. Organic scraps from the kitchen can also be placed inside this compost bin.

Thermophilic bacteria (bacteria that thrive in heat) drive the process of converting human waste to compost. They live in human feces, animal manure and compost heaps and generally prefer environments with a temperature of 108–150°F. The great benefit to this type of composting is that the heat kills the pathogenic microbes found in human waste that prefer cooler conditions, namely the average body temperature, 98°F.

Factory-made Composting Toilet

If you have a spare thousand dollars, you can purchase the best human waste disposal device money can buy, the factory-made composting toilet. This is the most trouble-free and green method of waste disposal available. Most are used by people who live in rural areas that do not have running water, and they are also used by many environmentalists. The best have no odors, look similar to real toilets, and can be placed inside the home. The most popular companies that manufacture these toilets are Envirolet (www.envirolet.com), Clivus Multrum Composting Toilet Systems (www.clivusmultrum.com), and Sun Frost composting toilets (www.sunfrost.com/composting_toilets.html).

CHAPTER 12

Lighting, Power and Heating

AS A SMALL CHILD I EXPERIENCED THE FAMOUS BLACKOUT OF 1965, THE BIG ONE THAT knocked out the electricity for New York City, most of the Northeast and even a small part of Canada. I was sitting in the backseat of my father's Studebaker as we slowly made our way home on the Major Deegan Expressway, looking back at a city covered in darkness.

My next blackout, in 1977, wasn't nearly as widespread, but a thousand times more chaotic. Pandemonium struck New York City for 25 hours when everything shut down in the middle of a heat wave and a major economic recession. In these volatile conditions the inner city erupted: over 2,000 stores were looted, nearly 4,000 arrests were made, and property damage was estimated at over $1 billion. Mayor Abe Beame called it "New York's night of terror." Like the blackout of '65, this one had a simple cause. A lightning strike at a power relay station triggered multiple system failures.

Twenty-six years later on August 1, 2003, I experienced the "mother of all blackouts" when over 50 million people in eight states and the Province of Ontario, Canada had their power wiped out. An official American-Canadian task force blamed the largest blackout in North American history on the failure of an Ohio power company to trim a few trees. On September 12, 2005, another small accident triggered by a Los Angeles electrical worker blacked out the entire city for a few hours. If you can draw one conclusion from all these incidents, it would be that our nation has a fragile, antiquated and unstable power grid that can easily be crippled by small accidents. If a clumsy electrician can shut off lights for 50 million people, what could a terrorist do?

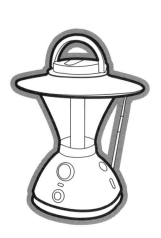
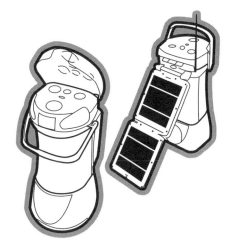

Hand-Crank Lantern　　　　**SL9000 Solar Rechargeable Lantern**

This is why you must begin to take the necessary steps that will prepare you to face the next power emergency whether it is accidental or deliberate. Blackouts don't just shut down your lights and television. They are serious technological emergencies that disrupt communications, transportation, medical services, food storage and more. A large disaster can shut down power for long periods. If you want the ability to comfortably ride them out, you will need safe, reliable and relatively inexpensive emergency lighting and power generation equipment.

Keeping lights on during power outages is a relatively simple task. All you need is a reliable source of light along with a power source. The best and easiest method is to use an electric camping lantern. It is durable, can be moved anywhere, and most can burn continuously for four hours or more. One of my favorite emergency lamps is the Global Marketing Technologies' SL9000 Solar Lantern—a solar rechargeable 9-watt mini powerhouse capable of illuminating a good-sized room. I also like the SL9100 Navigator. It is very thin, pivots, and can burn for seven hours on high. Both are available at 21st-century-goods.com.

Coleman manufactures durable battery-powered lanterns, as do Eveready, Garrett, and B-Solar. The Wonder-Lite Lantern includes an AM-FM radio with a hand crank that can be used to recharge its battery or power it during operation. Always remember to buy extra fluorescent light bulbs for the lanterns.

The batteries that you choose are equally important. Rechargeable types are best. They are costlier than ordinary disposable types, but they are indispensable during emergencies because they allow you to reuse them hundreds of times. If you use rechargeable batteries in your flashlights or radios, you need two sets per each device. This will allow you to recharge each set by rotating them after use. Make certain that the second set is fully charged.

Next item on your emergency lighting list should be a solar battery charger. This will allow you to keep the batteries fully powered. If you can afford $150, I suggest that you purchase a high-speed solar charger like the types offered by Power Film. This solar cell can be rolled up and placed practically anywhere. This feature makes it portable and easy to use. If you live in a large city tenement or high-rise, you can attach them to anything exposed to direct sunlight for three hours and more. They can even be hung out of a window!

The Power Film solar chargers come in five, ten, twenty, thirty, and sixty watt sizes. I suggest nothing smaller than a 10-watt unit; the extra power they draw from sunlight will allow your batteries to charge faster. If you choose the Power Film system, you will also need the charging accessory called the RA-4. This unit can charge AA, AAA, C, D and 9V batteries. For more information about Power Film products, go to www.iowathinfilm.com.

Inpower 3-Way Solar Battery Charger, $49.99 (www.target.com).

An alternative option for emergency lighting would be a kerosene or butane powered lantern. Their only drawback is that they need flammable fuel to operate, but are otherwise good options. Coleman, Petromax, and Dietz all make excellent emergency kerosene and gas lanterns. I prefer using electric-powered lights to avoid having to use flammable fuels. In careless hands flammable fuel models can be dangerous. In addition, fuel is difficult to find during long-term emergencies.

Candle lanterns are fantastic lighting tools for power outages. They do not require flammable fuel (only candle refills), are weather-resistant, can produce a decent amount of light, and most can burn for 8-10 hours continuously. Some can be fitted with citronella candles to keep mosquitoes under control if you are stuck outdoors in the summertime, or with aromatherapy candles to help you get through a stressful situation. My favorite models are the Uco Candlelier and the REI and EMS Candle Lanterns, all available at www.REI.com and www.EMS.com. They don't produce as much light as the electric or kerosene lamps but they will not fail, will provide usable light and are the most cost-effective of all the illumination methods listed.

A hardcore method of creating an emergency candle lantern is to take a regular aluminum soda can, use a very sharp knife or scissors to cut a very straight line at the center of the can from the top to bottom. Then make a 2" cut along the top and bottom rim of the can in both directions. Once that is done, carefully (the edges are sharp!) take the cut sections and open them wide like two doors. Light a small candle and let the wax drip at the bottom of the can to make a solid base for the candle. Place the candle inside at the center of the can. Pull up the tab of the can so it is pointing straight up. The open sections act as reflectors to amplify the light. Just make sure not to place the can near any flammable material or objects because the lit candle can be knocked out by a strong jolt.

If you require more light, you will need a system that can generate power.

If you live in an apartment, emergency power generation is tricky. Gas-powered generators cannot be used because of the volatility of the gasoline and the potentially lethal carbon monoxide exhaust fumes. High-tech methods to generate indoor power (such as hydrogen fuel cells and thermophotoelectric generators) are still being tested by manufacturers and will not be available to consumers for years.

The only safe, reliable, and simple method of emergency electrical power generation available to you is solar. In some limited cases, wind power. With a few adjustments and adaptations in your home, you can use solar modules and small wind turbines for emergency electrical power generation in practically any living environment that has a decent amount of sunlight or wind. A system of this type will generate just enough electrical energy to charge a 12V deep-cycle battery. When combined with a device called a power inverter (this changes DC current into AC), you can use it to run small energy-saving lights, a radio, small TV, or even a small portable refrigerator—this is especially important for diabetics, for whom insulin must be kept refrigerated. Many people around the world are embracing this method of power generation. They are setting up small power generation systems in unlikely places like apartment buildings, small businesses and other environments. They even have a name—Solar Guerrillas. Here is their manifesto:

> *We hold these truths to be self-evident, that all energy is freely and democratically provided by Nature, that utilities both public and private*

have no monopoly on the production and distribution of energy, that this century's monopolization of energy by utilities threatens the health of our environment and the very life of our planet.

We, the Solar Guerrillas of this planet, therefore resolve to place energy made from sunshine, wind, and falling water on this planet's utility grids with or without permission from utilities or governments.

We resolve to share this energy with our neighbors without regard for financial compensation.

We further resolve that our renewable energy systems will be safe and will not harm utility workers, our neighbors, or our environment.

I have been a Solar Guerrilla for over a decade. This allows me to know how to set up practical solar power systems in nearly any environment. If you decide to use a solar emergency power generation system, you should join our ranks. A great way to begin learning some Solar Guerrilla tips is to purchase a subscription to *Home Power Magazine* (contact subscription@homepower.com).

Check out this link to view some examples of effective solar power setups: www.homepower.com/magazine/guerrilla.cfm.

Emergency solar– and wind–powered systems vary in their size and output. A basic emergency solar power system consists of the photovoltaic module (solar cell), which converts sunlight into electrical energy; the storage battery to hold this energy; and the inverter.

A basic emergency wind-powered battery recharging system would consist of:

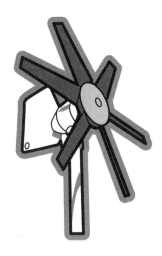

- The turbine.
- A steel mast to hold the turbine. Water pipes, old fence poles, or scaffold tubing will do.
- Guy wire (galvanized steel wire) to keep the system steady in high winds.
- Mounting brackets.
- Tensioners (small turnbuckle devices used to add tension to wire).
- 12V DC deep cycle battery.
- Voltage regulator.
- Fuses.
- Ammeter (measures electric current in amperes).
- Electrical wire.

Ampair Wind Turbine

Wind-powered battery recharging systems are in some ways less complex than their solar counterparts. If you live in a fairly windy city, such as Chicago, a small turbine mounted on a rooftop will supply just enough current to keep batteries charged. If your landlord permits it, a wind-powered battery can be mounted on your roof or fire escape. Suitable wind turbines for the city are the Ampair Hawk and the Southwest Windpower Air 403.

Many companies offer portable emergency solar power systems that are inexpensive and easy to use. Light-collecting modules must be placed where exposure to sunlight is maximized. This could be on your roof or outside your windows (mounted like satellite dishes).

If these emergency power systems won't give you enough energy, and you have the means and rights, you should seriously consider setting up a complete solar power system. This is expensive and sometimes legally difficult, but you will never see another electric bill, so the system will eventually pay for itself. Solar-only pioneers usually own the buildings they live in, since most buildings must be modified to accommodate solar power.

When There Is No Sun or Wind

If you live in a basement or other area with little or no sunlight and wind, or cannot afford a wind- or solar-powered system, you can still pursue other methods of emergency power generation. Only serious survivalists travel down this route, but maybe you are ready and willing to go totally hardcore, *i.e.,* to use a hand-crank or pedal-powered generator. Some military surplus stores occasionally sell old military hand-crank units, but they are hard to find. You might have to build one from scratch. Guidance is available from many sources; for example, the February/March 2001 issue of *Home Power* featured an article about a great system built by Aaron Dahlen.

Diesel and Gas Generators for Emergency Home Power

If you own your own house, you have the option of using a gas or diesel generator. Gas generators are more commonly used for home emergency power systems, because of the availability of gasoline and their low cost, ease of use, and variety.

Although diesel fuel isn't as readily available as gasoline, the generators are much more durable, better at handling larger loads, and able to run on alternative fuels such as vegetable oil. Fuel costs for diesel generators are lower than for gasoline ones, and they need less maintenance.

Base your choice of generator on the following criteria:

- The size of the electrical load in your home. Base this figure on the power required to operate only essential appliances such as refrigerators, lights, communications devices, water pumps, peripheral items in your heating system (fans), and some power tools. Include computers if you consider Internet access essential.
- Durability, ease of operation and maintenance, and spare parts availability. Do not purchase an engine manufactured in China, or any generic brand generator, unless you have direct access to spare parts and technical support.
- Whether you need prime or standby power. Prime power is for when you have no other power source available, and standby power is a backup for your local utility company. Most people in the U.S. only need standby power systems, but some in rural areas, hardcore survivalists and people who live off-grid (deliberately detached from utility lines) need prime power systems. Mini battery-powered standby power systems can be improvised, but only by people who have experience working with batteries, inverters and other electrical equipment. *The American Survival Guide* (now *Modern Survival Magazine,* www.modernsurvival.net), offered a great emergency power system in its January 2000 issue. This system, designed by Jeffrey D. Madeira, who runs a company called Systems Integration Specialists, produces 12V DC current and 120V AC.
- When diesel is a feasible option: a four-cycle industrial liquid-cooled diesel engine is best. They are less noisy and need less maintenance, exhaust venting, filters, and mufflers.
- Your power requirements. If you do not operate any devices (such as construction-grade power tools) that require more than 4 horsepower, you will only need a generator that produces single-phase (120/240V) power. Otherwise, you probably need triple-phase (120/208V–277/480V).

Emergency Cooking for the Home

During power service disruptions, you will need to have a emergency cooking method. This will require an emergency stove that can be used indoors safely. The simplest and least expensive type is a folding camp stove that works with your emergency candles (Nuwick) from your Grab-and-Go Bag. Using the extra wicks that come with the candles, a folding stove can boil about one quart of water in 10 to 12 minutes (depending on the ambient air temperature and

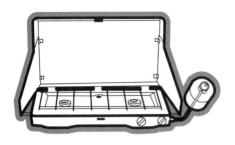

Coleman Folding Camp Stove

altitude). A few notches higher in their emergency value are multi-fuel back-packing stoves. The best I have used are the Optimus hiker's stoves and the Primus Vari-Fuel LFS. They can boil over 16 ounces of water in less than three minutes (at sea level, outdoors, with low wind). They use practically any type of fuel—alcohol, kerosene, diesel, and even spirits. These stoves can be found at EMS (www.EMS.com) and REI (www.REI.com).

I also like the Sierra stove. This is a small (one lb.) backpacker's stove that uses twigs, pinecones, bark as fuel. The Sierra stove uses a forced ventilation system (a battery-powered fan) to produce intense heat (18,000BTU/hr) enough to boil a quart of water in four minutes.

Propane emergency stoves are safer to use, as long as you store the compressed fuel cans in a safe and cool place. Coleman makes an excellent two-burner stove that can boil about a quart of water in five minutes. It can be placed atop your range and used like a regular stove until your power is restored, as long as you have enough fuel cans. Use these types of stove only in a well-ventilated area. The burning fuel can quickly and silently fill a room with toxic carbon monoxide gas.

Emergency Heat

To prepare for cold-weather emergencies when your usual source of heat becomes unavailable, begin by checking your home for cracks and gaps where warm air can escape and cold air enters. Caulk them up and make sure to install weather stoppers under every door. Then get an emergency heat source that does not produce toxic emissions (carbon monoxide), is sturdily constructed, stable and UL-tested. Your choice should take into account the particulars of your living space.

Kerosene heaters are relatively inexpensive, efficient heating units of two types, vented (with external fuel tanks) and unvented (with fuel tanks

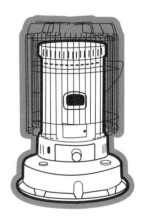

Kerosene Heater

attached to the unit). Homeowners can use the vented type. Apartment dwellers must use unvented heaters, because of a lack of space and fire safety concerns. But unvented kerosene space heaters produce dangerous fumes and therefore require a lot of ventilation. To operate one safely, you would need to keep your windows open, an obviously inefficient setup.

Electric space heaters are less expensive and do not produce fumes, but electricity may not be available during an emergency. If you choose to purchase an electric space heater, make sure that it has an on-off indicator light, an automatic shut-off switch for when the unit is knocked over, and a long cord. Plug it directly into the wall—do not use extension cords or overload the outlet.

Gas heaters are the cleanest-burning fuel-consuming devices. They do not need venting or electricity (unless you purchase a model with a blower). Most people, however, do not have a safe place to store large quantities of propane.

Worst-Case Situation Heating

To endure protracted crises, you will need to consider another method of keeping your home warm. The only sure-fire emergency heating device that does not require specially prepared and volatile fuel is the wood-burning stove. Tens of thousands of Russians survived by using wood-burning stoves during winter 2002–2003. Across the country, old and poorly maintained water pipes and boilers burst, leaving many people without heat and hot water during one of the coldest winters in decades.

Old rolled-up newspapers, clothing, and other materials were burned for life-saving heat in the -30 degrees Celsius environment. For many Russians, knowing how to safely heat their homes with this type of stove saved them from hypothermia, frostbite, or death.

Worst-Case Situation Emergency Apartment Heating

A modified "Four Dog" or **trail stove** can heat your home, food, and water. A company called Four Dog Stoves (www.fourdog.com) manufactures a number of great models including a lightweight titanium model.

- Before installing the stove, select an area close to a window for the stovepipe and vent.
- All flammable material must be moved away from the unit.
- Keep a mid-sized ABC fire extinguisher nearby on a wall mount.

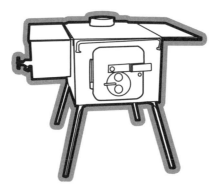

Four Dog Stove

- Do not put the stove where it blocks an exit.
- If you have children, erect a barrier around the stove to keep them from the hot surfaces.
- Remove the curtains from the window with the stovepipe air vent. Besides the stove, you will need the following:
- 90-degree elbow joint (to be attached at the top of the stovepipe, to direct it).
- Stovepipe extensions and adapter.
- Heat shields for any surfaces within 36 inches of the stove.
- Carbon monoxide detectors.

Safe operation of an emergency wood stove requires many modifications. If your idea of power tools is a new piece of software, hire a professional to get the job done right. A poorly installed or unsafely operated wood stove can jeopardize the safety of your family and everyone in your building.

For further reading:

The Complete Book of Heating with Wood by Larry Gay (Storey Publishing, 1974).

Jay Shelton's Solid Fuel Encyclopedia, by Jay W. Shelton (Garden Way Publishing Company, 1982).

Fireplaces and Chimneys (Farmers' Bulletin No. 1889), U.S. Department of Agriculture. Government Printing Office.

Woodburner's Companion by Dirk Thomas (Allan C. Hood and Co., 2000).

CHAPTER 13

Emergency Communication

TEMPORARY COMMUNICATIONS DISRUPTIONS IN LARGE CITIES ARE MORE COMMON THAN YOU might think. They may result from power outages, fires, or other frequently encountered urban technological problems. But when major disasters strike, the damaged communication lines may require many days to repair broken equipment and restore regular service. Your cellular phone service can also be disrupted.

Prepare yourself and your loved ones for a communications breakdown by discussing the possibility in advance and make a plan of action in case you are separated when the breakdown occurs. It is critical that everyone in your house has filled out their own Emergency Escape Location Card (E.E.L. Card) in advance (see page 167 for E.E.L. Card description), and keep it with them at all times. If anyone is unable to come home, when disaster strikes, you will already have alternate locations specified at which to meet.

The only way to effectively communicate over long distances during communication system failures is by two-way radio transmitters. The best types to own for emergency use are walkie-talkies, as they are easy to use and portable. There are many different types available today. The most practical units for regular folks are:

General Mobile Radio Service (GMRS) Radios

These have an operating range from 5–25 miles. The GMRS service was created by the Federal Communications Commission to provide families with a reliable form of short-distance communications that can be used during outings. To operate GRMS units, you need to file for an FCC license.

FRS (Family Radio Service) Radios

Family Radio Service band "walkie-talkies" have become quite popular the past few years. They are an inexpensive way to keep in touch with family members or friends over short distances (about four city blocks or one to three miles in an open rural area). They are especially useful during emergencies when you need to keep in touch around large crowds and confusion. You don't need a license for FRS radios, but the FCC does have a strict set of rules regarding their use (i.e., you can't use foul language or make any modifications on your radio and you cannot monitor other people's transmissions).

Hand-held ham units are able to communicate over long distances. The radio-to-radio range of a small five-watt output hand-held ham radio can vary depending on sunspot activity, your location and a few other factors. Hand-held ham units can also bounce signals off radio signal regenerators called "repeaters," that can significantly extend their operational range. To own and operate a ham radio, you must first get a basic FCC "no-code" technician class license. "No-code" means that you will not have to learn Morse code to use a system. You will also need to take a relatively simple 35-question multiple-choice test. If you pass your test, your class of license will allow you to access different ham frequencies above 30 megahertz (MHz).

High quality GMRS and FRS radios range in price from $50–$150 per pair and Motorola, Cobra and Uniden make great models. Some of the best hand-held ham units available are manufactured by Motorola, Yaesu and Kenwood. Extra performance comes with a price. Hand-held ham radios are costlier than GMRS and FRS counterparts. If you want an extra edge in an emergency and are willing to learn how to use them properly they are worth the extra cash.

IA TIP

The detonation of a nuclear weapon can produce an enormous electromagnetic pulse (called EMP for short). If you are within range of the detonation, the massive electrical charge released can disable your hand held digital radios. The only way to prevent this from occurring is if you improvise a device called a Faraday Cage. This is a metal box or screen that can absorb the EMP.

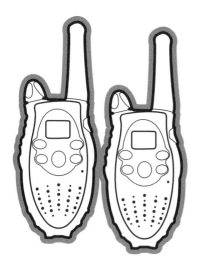

You can build an improvised Faraday Cage or pouch with metal mesh found at most hardware stores. You could also find a metal box in which you can stow your radios. Get some foam rubber and make a sleeve to keep the radio in a fixed position. If a nuke is ever detonated, the electrical charge produced by the EMP will be absorbed by the metal, which will protect the radio's circuitry. You can use this method to protect all sensitive electrical equipment.

Motorola FRS Radios

Radio Scanners

Another valuable and relatively affordable communications tool is a radio scanner. Once programmed by the user, this device will automatically scan over and lock onto different radio frequencies used by police, the military and other responders who are called out to service during emergencies. Having the ability to listen in on their conversations provides you with important information that may help you during a crisis or disaster.

Uniden makes excellent hand-held units that are easy to use, and many are reasonably priced. You will need some reference material to teach you the ins and outs about the proper use of scanners and different active frequencies. The book Scanners and Secret Frequencies by Harry Eisenson is a great place to start.

Emergency communications is such a detailed and important a topic, it would be good to follow up on its study. Guide to Emergency Survival Communications by Dave Ingram gives you a detailed look at all of the things that you need to know about this very important subject.

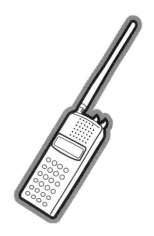

Uniden Radio Scanner

CHAPTER 14

Evacuation Protocols

A LARGE DISASTER MAY PRODUCE CONDITIONS THAT REQUIRE YOU TO RAPIDLY EVACUATE FROM your home, office, or immediate area. To avoid confusion, you must construct an emergency evacuation plan before the disaster strikes.

Advance Planning Is Crucial

- Before an emergency strikes, pre-select the method of travel and the first location that you will evacuate to. Ask local authorities in advance about emergency evacuation routes. Choose alternates in case the area of your first choice is compromised by hazardous conditions created by the emergency.
- Contact your local Red Cross and Salvation Army and collect as much information as you can about emergency evacuation shelter locations in or near your community. Include this in your plan.
- Take note of where hospitals, police, gas stations, and water are located in proximity to your path.
- Make a list of potential hazards, detours or obstacles you may encounter along each route and make appropriate contingency plans for each situation.
- Finally, identify each evacuation route that you choose to utilize in your area and travel along it to the planned destination. You should create a few of your own special personal routes as well.

The best evacuation plans are prepared by you well before the disaster strikes—and *never* in its midst. It is also vital to know what types of disasters provoke emergency evacuations. Knowing this will help you to make the proper judgment call if you find yourself caught in a situation where you believe a rapid evacuation may be required. In some limited cases, immediate evacuation during or after the disaster may not be necessary or even prudent if you don't have the proper PPEs (Personal Protective Equipment) and reliable methods of transportation. You could place yourself in even greater danger by exposing yourself to disaster-related hazards such as falling or collapsing debris (earthquakes), dangerous chemicals (toxic gas chemical/biological weapons release), fallout (as in a nuclear emergency) and other dangers.

If you live in or near an area that has frequent tornadoes or other weather-related disasters, keep your ears open for sirens. If you want to be extra safe, purchase a radio scanner or radio that receives the NOAA weather band. See www.nws.noaa.gov/nwr/indexnw.htm. You will find the frequency for all U.S. counties. During tornado season, keep your radio on and stay alert at all times.

Staying Informed Before and After You Leave

As we saw in New Orleans and Texas, after hurricanes Katrina and Rita, evacuation information from your local authorities or other officials can be inaccurate, confusing and even dangerous. Many of the evacuation plans currently in place are at best quite shaky—at worst, totally ineffective.

You are better off paying close attention to your local TV and radio news. They have reporters on the ground and in the air who will provide you with more reliable information. Still, if you have a radio scanner, make sure to look up the broadcasting frequencies of the local authorities in your area and keep it turned on and tuned in, so you can hear what they're communicating to each other. You should also familiarize yourself with the most important emergency codes the police use to identify trouble. This is so you can understand what they are saying when they speak in code to each other. You can look up police codes here: www.radiolabs.com/police-codes.htm.

When used properly, a scanner can be one of your most important survival tools. Common sense helps, too. If you hear something that doesn't sound quite right, don't react until you analyze the details and weigh your best options for a successful outcome. See Chapter 11 for communication options while on the road.

Before you leave your home or business...

- Disconnect all electrical appliances, TV and tools. Turn off electrical power at the junction box and gas at the main valve. Don't attempt to shut down any electrical devices if you are wet or standing in floodwater.
- Tighten all the gas caps on your vehicles and heating fuel tanks to minimize seepage if they are submerged.
- If you are entering a flood situation, place your Grab-and-Go Bag inside three large heavy-duty trash bags. Make certain that all sharp objects are packed away deep inside the Grab-and-Go Bag. Blow air into the bags and tie the bags tightly at the top to form an airtight seal. Wrap

a strong thick cord around the knot at the top and tie a tether line to your waist. The bag should float, and you can drag it through the waters behind you.

■ Don't forget your cash. During large evacuations, you may not be able to use your credit cards or withdraw money from an ATM. This is why it is necessary to carry emergency money at all times—enough to help you pay for transportation, supplies or whatever you may need to get to a safe area. You should carry it in a small belt pouch—or even a money belt to protect it from loss or theft.

IA TIP

Keep your emergency money sacred. Never spend it unless you absolutely have to. Running short of cash during a trip to the grocery store does not fall into the emergency category. Each member of your family should carry emergency money—except children under 12, unless they are very responsible.

Evacuating the Area

If you have a family or loved ones, you will need a sure-fire method that will allow you to keep track of each person's movements and to know where they will be—in case you are separated and the communications systems fail. I created the E.E.L. card for just this purpose.

How to Use an Emergency Escape Location Card (E.E.L.)

E.E.L.s provide a way to find lost family members during emergency evacuations. Give an E.E.L. card to each member of your family (or friends) whom you wish to keep track of during a communications breakdown.

■ Select a number of emergency evacuation meeting locations or areas.
■ You will need one E.E.L. card per location per person.
■ Make a list of each emergency evacuation location point—starting from first evacuation point to last. Five locations are usually more than enough.

Choose multiple evacuation locations because your first selected area may be compromised by hazardous conditions, damage or another dangerous situation. Or you may not be able to reach the location because of travel restrictions. The extra choices allow you to move to alternative areas if your original choices are compromised or unsafe.

- Write the address or area of your first meeting point underneath the words *E.E.L. Address Number One.*
- Include specific details about the chosen location, especially if it is in unfamiliar territory. Example: "2745 Cherry Tree Rd., Apt. 5H—two doors down from the large fire-station, look for broken sign in front."
- If further detail is needed, use the grid in the small box on the right side of the card to draw a small map of the location or meeting area.
- If the location has a phone number, include it. The last line has space for two or three more additional emergency numbers.
- After the word "Start", fill in the time you will begin checking the location for your family and/or friends. In the blank after, fill in when you will end checking for the day. At "Frequency", fill in how frequently you will return to the site during the time span specified.

Another accuracy measure built into the E.E.L. cards: you can also list the days that you will check the meeting spot. It may take more than a few hours to rendezvous' with family members. The severity of the emergency may not permit them to move freely for the first few days.

Family members or friends can even prepare special E.E.L. cards that will allow them to locate each other even under the worst conditions. These would contain specific instructions and details about the locations where the group or individuals meet. For example, an E.E.L. card might contain information that specifies where the nearest hospital or police station is in proximity to the emergency meeting point. It could also include the nearest pay phone, water source, shelter, etc.

To make your own E.E.L. card, make a copy from the back of this book or go to www.PreparednessNow.net and download and print a copy. Fill in your information, reduce it to the whatever size suits you, then laminate it to prevent it from falling apart, or the ink wearing off. I recommend punching a hole at the top, and fastening your cards together with a key ring string or twist tab. Carry the cards with you at all times.

EMERGENCY EVACUATION CARD

Address 1 _2745 Cherry Tree Road_
Apt. 5H
_555-1234_
Address 2 _7623 Lamanda Ave._
_555-2946_

Start _10_ (AM) _6_ (AM)
Frequency _hourly_
Days _M-F_
Start _2_ (PM) _7_ (PM)
Frequency _half-hour_
Days _sat & sun_

Locations _Two doors from the fire station_

Emergency Telephone Numbers _555-5678 Grandma June_

EMERGENCY EVACUATION CARD

Notes
_Tim Jones lives next door
in Apt. 7H (555-9876)_

Alternate Locations
_Library down the street
from fire station_

Fire Station

Emergency Evacuation Steps

If you are not separated from your family and are at home, gather together your Grab-and-Go Bag, handcart, and other important gear.

Check your radio for critical information about emergency shelter, food, water and transportation. The EAS (Emergency Alert Systems) will inform you about safe evacuation routes and the location of Red Cross Emergency shelters/registration centers. Once you are checked in to a center, your relatives and friends will also have a way to track you down. You should also have a map of your city so you can move through unfamiliar areas quickly and easily without getting lost.

If you can afford it, and don't mind carrying the extra gear, you can purchase a hand-held GPS (Global Positioning System) device. This can help you to navigate through unfamiliar territory without a map.

If you have a large Grab-and-Go Bag, use your handcart to move it. It is important to conserve energy during an evacuation.

Make sure to wear your most comfortable and durable clothing. A great garment to have for an evacuation is a fisherman's vest. Fisherman's vests have large and small pockets for frequently used small items. Cabelas.com has one of the largest selections. The larger Civilian Lab models such as the Covert Specialist will also serve you well. They have many internal pockets and their design allows for very easy access.

Wear sturdy, comfortable shoes—you will be spending a great deal of time in them during a forced evacuation. You should make the shoes as comfortable as you can by using cushions (Sorbothane are best), arches, or whatever else is needed to make them comfortable. I believe that steel-toed work boots with ankle support are best despite their added weight because they provide protection from sharp metal objects, glass and other hazards that could produce a serious foot wound. It goes without saying that a foot injury during an evacuation can significantly slow your escape.

If you are in an area with damaged structures, falling debris will be a threat. Wear a protective helmet if you included it in your Grab-and-Go Bag. A bicycle helmet would be better than nothing.

Keep your eyes and head covered—you don't want to deal with an eye injury during emergency evacuation.

Pre-select relatives or friends that live outside your immediate area as a central contact for family members to get information about your location and condition. Remember that this can only work when telephone services are functioning.

If you are evacuating during a nuclear or biological emergency, wear protective clothing over your regular clothing. Remember to put your Grab-and-Go Bag and any other extra gear inside large plastic garbage bags sealed tight. Use three bags to be on the safe side, and seal them up with duct or gaffers tape.

If you do not have any protective clothing, wear a raincoat or windbreaker. Use a hat (or helmet) to cover your head, and a dust mask to cover your nose. If you do not have goggles, improvise a pair to protect your eyes. In a nuclear emergency, you must limit your exposure to fallout and move to the nearest shelter as quickly as possible. To know about radiation levels, you will need to own a detection device such as the NukAlert (see Chapter 20) or some other type of radiation detection device.

Animals will not be allowed inside most emergency shelters and will need to be left at home during forced evacuations. The only way that you will be able to keep your pet is if you travel to your destination on foot or by personal vehicle. If you bring your pet, you will need to carry extra food, water and plastic bags to dispose of their waste.

If you own a dog, you must leave at home and purchase an auto feeder and automatic water system in case the worst happens. Epets.com sells a six-day automatic pet feeder and a five-gallon capacity automatic water bowl. This type of system can sustain a medium-sized pet for up to one month.

If you have children in school, make sure to leave information with the teacher or principal regarding family members (or friends) who are authorized to pick up your children in case of emergency. If possible, provide pictures of the individuals so no mistakes can be made.

If you are traveling with an infant or toddler, bring extra clothing, children's medicine (Motrin, Tylenol), baby soap, lotion, blankets and as many baby wipes as you can carry.

Elderly and Physically Challenged Emergency Evacuation

If you are elderly or physically challenged you will need to make special preparations for an emergency evacuation. You will need support. You must have a home care attendant, nurse, family members or friends that are ready, willing and able to assist you during this difficult period. This helper will need to be physically fit enough to move and lift you across, over, or around obstacles that you may encounter along the evacuation route—in my experience, it would take two people or more to safely move an immobile elderly or injured person during a mass evacuation.

If you need special equipment such as wheelchairs, walkers, oxygen tanks, battery powered nebulizers and other forms of medical gear, you must have portable versions that can be more easily transported. Elderly or ill evacuees must have all of their primary medications packed and ready to travel to ensure that if a disaster strikes, the help would not waste time searching for it.

If the emergency involves nuclear, chemical or biological material, the appointed helper will need to have proper protective gear that corresponds with the specific emergency. They will also need to know how to properly use the equipment.

Deaf evacuees will need someone that can alert them to an emergency if they are asleep. Vibrating emergency beepers are useful in this regard. Blind evacuees will need reliable guides that can help them to a safe area or assistance.

A special evacuation plan for evacuees with special needs should be prepared to include emergency escape routes that bypass large hills, staircases and rough terrain.

Remember to carry energy-producing "trail foods" that you can snack on while moving. Nuts, dried fruit and granola or jerky (meat or vegetarian) will help to keep your energy levels high. Try to carry with you at least one gallon of drinking water. It is crucial to keep your body hydrated.

Emergency Evacuation by Inflatable Boat

If you own an inflatable boat like the one described in the following chapter on emergency transportation and live close to a large body of water, you can use it to evacuate to a safe area. Before you make your move, there are a few things that you must consider.

Do you have a pre-planned destination, and will you be able to get there from your present location? Do you have any experience in operating this type of boat and are you a strong swimmer in case the boat fails?

What will you do if your motor breaks down? Do you have oars that allow you to row the boat? Are you fit enough to row a fully loaded boat for a long period? If your boat uses a gas powered motor, do you have enough fuel? If you have an electric motor, are the batteries fully charged? What is the range of the gas powered motor on a full tank with the boat fully loaded? The battery powered motor?

What is the maximum weight limit rating for your boat, and how much will you be loading it with? These are the primary questions you must ask yourself if you plan to use a small boat for an emergency evacuation.

Evacuations are one of the most stressful aspects of any emergency. In order to be properly prepared, one should take the time to conduct a practice drill. If you live in an area that has frequent emergencies like tornadoes, hurricanes or earthquakes, stage a drill often enough so that the procedures become routine.

CHAPTER 15

Emergency Transportation

IF YOU HAVE EVER BEEN STUCK IN A RUSH-HOUR TRAFFIC JAM IN A LARGE CITY, YOU'LL UNDER-stand the need for alternative transportation during disasters and emergencies. During working hours, the traffic speed in large cities averages between a slow crawl and a complete stop. Congestion is already a major problem, and a disaster will make it exponentially worse.

Bicycles

If you do not own a bicycle, get one—if not for recreational use, then for emergencies. Outside of walking, bicycles are the most reliable way of moving around during a crisis. During and after a major disaster, streets will likely be closed to civilian motor traffic to make room for emergency vehicles. Public transportation systems will be switched to limited service or temporarily halted. Side streets are likely to become clogged with heavy traffic.

A good bicycle will allow you to get around the traffic, and a bicycle can be carried over roadblocks or fallen debris. It's also possible to haul gear and supplies with the right accessories. And if you aren't in the best of shape, you can purchase small electric or gasoline bicycle motors to help reduce the workload.

Riding Through the Storm

Riding a bicycle during a disaster differs from recreational riding. Speeding fire trucks, police cars, ambulances and other emergency vehicles increase risk and the need for vigilance. Confusion and panic will drive crowds of people with their children and animals into the streets. In some cases, debris from buildings may litter the streets. Smoke from fires can impair vision and even restrict breathing. Bicycling in these conditions is difficult and perilous. The following tips will help reduce your risk.

- Use puncture-resistant tires (or airless tires) because a flat tire during or after a disaster could be a life-threatening inconvenience. Puncture-resistant tires are usually lined with Dupont Kevlar, the material of bulletproof vests. Airless tires use a polyurethane foam or a urethane elastomeric material. They are the best way to avoid having to change bicycle tires on busy city streets, and your bike will always be ready to roll. I have used Kevlar-lined tires to ride on broken glass-speckled streets of New York City and they haven't failed me yet.
- Strong rims are essential. A bent rim can restrict or even prevent riding, and rims are difficult to repair in transit, particularly for amateurs. Weak rims bend easily when you are riding over rugged terrain or carrying your Grab-and-Go Bag and other gear. You need a rim that can handle extra weight and rough terrain.

The strongest rims available are WTC Clincher Rims, which are 50% thicker than regular bike rims and have rolled edges and dimpled spoke-holes for added strength. They are made like motorcycle wheels and are practically impossible to bend, making them perfect wheels for an emergency bicycle.

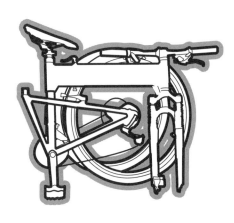

**Montague Paratrooper
Folding Bicycle**

Best Bike for Emergencies

My personal choice for emergency transportation and recreation is the Montague Paratrooper, which was designed for the military and is the best, most durable folding bicycle on the market. The Montague weighs less than 30 pounds and fits into a bag to be carried anywhere.

I have put this bike through the wringer, riding it all around New York City and Los Angeles, and on backwoods trails in New Mexico, Pennsylvania, and New York with up to 50 pounds of gear. It performs fantastically and has my vote for the best emergency transportation bicycle and city living.

Getting Ready to Ride

Using a bicycle during an emergency requires stamina, so it makes preparedness sense to ride the bike whenever possible. Bicycling is an excellent way to integrate your fitness plan with ordinary activities. Bad air quality makes an air filter mask an important piece of bike safety equipment.

Bicycle Motors

Bicycle motors reduce your workload. Bicycles equipped with electric or gas motors are the best and most reliable form of urban emergency transportation.

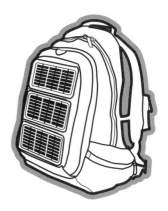

Electric motors require less maintenance than gasoline, and when you use rechargeable batteries and a photovoltaic trickle charger, you will never need to worry about finding gasoline.

The electric motor can be easily charged wherever you can find power; or, if you can afford it, you can buy a portable photovoltaic battery charger that would make your bike into an SPV (solar powered vehicle). If you want to

Voltaic Solar Backpack

be really clever, you could jury-rig an Iowa Thin Film (www.powerfilmsolar.com) flexible photovoltaic panel to your Grab-and-Go Bag to trickle-charge your battery while you ride. The R-15 300 model has grommet holes at the edges

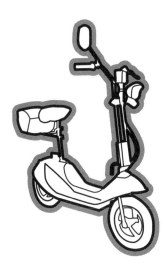

Xcooter Electric Scooter

of the panel, so you can tie it on. Or you can buy a backpack with solar modules and charging equipment built into the bag—Voltaic (www.voltaicsystems.com) makes one of the best available.

Pay close attention to the type of battery you choose to use. Lithium-ion polymer batteries are more expensive than lead-acid and nickel-metal hydride types but they are more powerful. One small ten-pound lithium-ion power pack is remarkably the equivalent of a large car battery.

A great gasoline motor for bikes is the Tecumseh Viper, a 2-horsepower, 2-stroke, 9-lb. wonder that can move a 200-pound man at 30 mph. Its 20-oz. gas tank powers a one-hour ride. Small gasoline motors, however, are temperamental and require maintenance to keep running at peak levels. But they provide more torque than most electric motors; if you are hauling heavy gear, bike motors take a lot of strain off your body, especially if you're going uphill.

All in all, bicycles equipped with electric or gas motors are the best and most reliable form of urban emergency transportation.

Mopeds, a gas-fed cross between a motorcycle, scooter and bicycle, is another great form of motorized emergency transportation. The best types of moped for emergency transportation have pedals, which allows for the option of riding them like a bicycle if the motor breaks down.

Some mopeds, like the TFR-USA can get up to 150 miles per gallon of gas (for a 220-lb. max load). This is a very important asset. A 150-mile range is more than enough to take you out of the danger area of nearly every sort of disaster.

IA TIP

Small gasoline engines require regular maintenance to work properly. If you have no mechanical skill, you should not purchase a gas powered bicycle motor or moped before you learn how to make some light repairs in the field.

Bike bags and bike racks help you carry your gear, and **trailer hitches** let you add anything you can tow. If you are strong and fit, you can move quite a bit of emergency gear this way. If you live in an area with extreme cold weather, you may need to ride through snow and ice, in which case you should consider studded bicycle tires such as those made by Nokian. There are also less expensive alternatives to buying studded tires. Cold-climate bicycling organizations such as the Edmonton (Canada) Bicycle Commuters (www.edmontonbicyclecommuters.ca) or (www.icebike.org) are good sources of information about how to customize a regular bike tire to travel over ice.

Alternatives to Bicycles

There are a few other excellent forms of emergency transportation to consider. Electric and gas-powered scooters are a great alternative to bikes. Scooters are easier to ride than motorcycles; anyone who can handle a bike can learn to ride one quickly, and they can also be used by people who aren't fit or strong enough to pedal around a disaster area. Their major limitations is that they need gas or a place to charge their batteries. In addition, most smaller gas-powered and electric scooters are unable to carry heavy loads or travel more than 20 miles at a time, and require more balance and skill to operate. They also cannot be used for anything other than a fancy chair if the motor breaks down.

Some smaller versions of motorized scooters are available that can be used as emergency escape vehicles. A company called Xcooter makes some great all-terrain gas- and electric- powered small scooters that are fast, durable, lightweight and small enough to pack in the trunk of a car.

Some regular human-powered scooters can also be used, provided that you live in an area that has paved roads, and are physically fit enough to ride around carrying a heavy Grab-and-Go Bag and other gear.

Emergency Boats

If you live near a large river or other body of water you might want to plan for emergency evacuation by small boat or raft. Some durable inflatable rafts, kayaks, and sport boats can be stored in a medium-sized closet. For example, Sea Eagle (www.seaeagle.com) makes an inflatable boat, the 14SR Sport runabout, that can carry seven adults and accommodate a 40-horsepower motor. If you live in an apartment without a safe area like a garage to store gasoline, you must use a smaller and less powerful electric motor.

The batteries and motor will add 270–300 pounds toward the weight limit of the small vessel. A 5-hp motor should be able to move a family of four and all of their gear (about 750 lbs) at about 5 mph for up to 30 miles in calm water. Heavy-duty 12-volt, deep-cycle, sealed lead acid gel batteries rated for at least 95 ampere-hours are best for this type of electric boat. You may also want to obtain a solar charger.

Emergency Rural Transportation

If you live in the country, you are going to need a vehicle that is extremely reliable, tough, and easy and inexpensive to maintain. It must be up to the challenge of handling floods, snow and ice storms, extreme cold and heat along with several other conditions that are frequently encountered in rural areas. In most cases, a normal 4x4 truck will do the trick, but if you believe that you need more, you might consider purchasing a Rodedawg amphibious SUV (www.rodedawg.com). It is diesel-powered and can easily be converted over to biofuel. The Rodedawg is designed to navigate crowded highways and swollen rivers without strain.

If you already have a truck, you could also consider investing in a camping trailer to sleep inside. If it is a full sized flatbed, consider the Quickup camper (www.quickupcamper.com), designed by industrial designer Jay Baldwin, a former Bucky Fuller student. Its design can be described as uplifting—literally! It folds down into a streamlined package and lifts up to create a wonderful mobile living space.

If you can't afford that, a tailgate tent will also do the trick. Your vehicle must also have its own Grab-and-Go bag built around the size and needs of your family, along with a spare tire, jack, flares, and tools, plus critical replacement parts (fan belts, spark plugs, etc.). You'll also need to keep an emergency supply of gas or diesel fuel in a large fuel tank that must be buried in a gravel bed on your property, along with a hand-powered pump to get the fuel.

Sci-Fi Emergency Transportation

Personal mini-helicopters will soon be widely available. Promising models include the Air Scooter, Solo Trek, and Gen H-4. These choppers range in price between $25,000 and $50,000, require no license to fly, and are sure to become popular among rich adventurers, police, and rescue workers. The Air Scooter stands out by including pontoons for water landings, a sturdy bicycle-like frame, and computer-free flight stabilization.

Dr. Paul Moeller has been working on his Skycar for nearly 40 years, and its commercial debut is projected for 2008. When the Skycar is finally for sale, it will be the ultimate emergency escape vehicle.

Over time, nontraditional vehicles such as these may become the norm. Until then, choose a system that is within your budget and suited to where you live and where you need to go in the event of a disaster. Get something together, even if it is only a plan. Your emergency transportation system will help you get away from trouble fast with your important gear to ride out the emergency more comfortably. Forced relocation is traumatic enough without having to struggle to move. A good emergency transportation system is worth every bit of time, money, and sweat that you put into it.

CHAPTER 16

Subway Escape

DURING AN EMERGENCY, AN URBAN SUBWAY MAY BE A DANGEROUS LOCATION. YOU ARE locked inside a steel container underground with narrow exit doors. One of the worst-case examples occurred on February 18, 2003 in Daegu, South Korea in which 196 people were killed by a fire set off inside a crowded subway car by an emotionally disturbed man. Passing trains fanned the flames and the doomed train car soon became a hurtling crematorium.

The subway platform can be hazardous, too. In an emergency evacuation, turnstiles and gates can restrict and sometimes stop movement altogether. Riders should take the following precautions when traveling on subways:

- Avoid crowds. The most dangerous time to ride the subway is during rush hour. Your chances of surviving a subway emergency increase significantly if you are riding in a car or waiting in a station with a smaller number of people than rush-hour crowds.
- While waiting on platforms, stand away from metal trash receptacles; a terrorist could place an explosive device inside to generate shrapnel when it is detonated.
- Stay close to an exit so you can get out of a station quickly in case of trouble. Your best chance of escaping subway trouble will depend upon how quickly you can gain access to an exit before crowds clog them up.
- If you ride the subway regularly, carry a flashlight (non-incendive) and a smoke escape hood. In a subway fire, the entire car or station can rapidly fill up with thick and toxic smoke that can overcome people in less than two minutes. Your smoke escape hood provides you with up to 15 minutes of breathable air. The extra time will allow you to use your flashlight to help you navigate your way out of the train, tunnel or station. If you do not have an escape hood, cover your nose and mouth with your shirt, scarf or tie. If you are carrying water, pour the water over the fabric before you press it to your face. This will buy you about one minute of extra time to move to a safer area before you pass out. Frequent subway riders are advised to carry their own smoke hood.

- Make sure to carry a mini-pry bar. Most modern subway trains use shatterproof lexan/glass windows that are very difficult to break through. A good mini-pry bar can help you to knock the window out of its setting, or even shatter it. You may also be able to use it if you need to break some of the small padlocks on other doors and gates.
- Familiarize yourself with all the exits at the stations that you frequently use. Suppose you need to get out of a subway station and the exit that you regularly use is blocked? Do you know where the other exits can be found, and quickly?
- Pay attention to the position of the train between stops. This information may be vital if you need to make an emergency evacuation from a stalled train in a tunnel. How close would you be to the next station stop? How far away would you be from the last? The closest station would be your best exit point.

To Help Determine Your Proximity to the Closest Station

- Be aware of the train's direction.
- Make a mental note of the approximate time it takes to travel between each station stop. With a little practice you will quickly know how to make accurate estimates of your approximate location between train stations. If you needed to evacuate the train, you'll be glad you paid attention.
- Learn about the hazards you would encounter during a rapid evacuation. For example, if you needed to move off a train quickly, you might have to step down onto the tracks near the "third rail," the subway train's power source. Third rails conduct enough current to fry you like a hamburger. You must know where it is, what it looks like and most importantly to keep away from it at all times while you are on the tracks. The third rail has a white cover plate in the New York City subway system. Switches, brake boxes, cables and conduit piping are another concern. In a dark

tunnel they can cause you to trip and fall. Exercise great caution and try not to fall out of sight of other evacuees.

- Try to spot where the emergency exits are located along your most frequently traveled subway routes. You can do this by scanning the tunnel outside the subway windows or asking subway employees.
- If you are a regular subway rider, carry work gloves in your E-Kit to protect your hands from injury in a possible evacuation.
- If you are a frequent subway rider, wear shoes that will allow you to walk comfortably on the track bed. An emergency may call for an evacuation, and high heels will not only make you uncomfortable, but could place your life in jeopardy in a dark subway tunnel filled with high voltage equipment.
- Be cautious of gas. During a subway mishap, pipes could be ruptured, releasing gas into the tunnel. This is why it is important to carry explosion-proof non-incendive flashlights.
- Listen to, and if possible stay close to, the subway conductor. They would likely be aware of the emergency exits; they also carry two-way radios that would be able to summon help.

How to Protect Yourself from a Chemical Weapons Release

In March 1995, the Om Shinrikyo cult group sent 12 members into Tokyo subway trains with six packages filled with deadly sarin nerve gas. They punctured the packages with umbrellas and released gas that rapidly filled the station and caused over 5,000 people to become violently ill. Twelve riders died.

Sarin is one of many different types of nerve agent that could be used by terrorists in a subway train or car. To protect yourself from nerve agents or other chemical weapons:

- Wear a shirt or jacket when you ride a subway or enter a crowded station. Nerve agents cause trouble through inhalation and skin absorption. If it is summertime, and you are wearing light clothing, purchase a light Gore-Tex windbreaker and carry it with you when you ride the subway.
- Carry your escape hood or P, N, or R 95-100 respirator masks if you regularly travel on a subway. If you begin to see crowds of people behaving unusually (rubbing eyes or coughing violently is the first indication of a chemical attack), quickly remove your escape hood or mask from its package, pull it on and rapidly (but calmly) move away from the area. Keep a cool head if you get caught in a large frightened crowd. Clothe your skin as much as possible, and when you

make it outside do not remove your clothing with your hands! Call for help from an EMT and warn them that you may have been exposed to a chemical agent before they touch you.

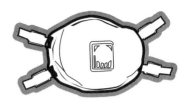

3M N100 Respirator Mask

- Move away from where the crowd is concentrated; explore alternative options for your exit from the station.
- If gas is released, passengers will begin to itch their eyes and cough and choke violently. You will only have a few seconds to move away from the area and put on your mask.
- If you travel with a stroller, you might want to carry an empty sturdy backpack or baby carrier. In the event of a crisis, the infant or small child can be placed snugly inside, leaving your hands free to help you maneuver.
- If the child is old enough, train them to put on an escape hood. I taught my three-year-old soon how to use his escape hood after the 9/11 attack, and he picked it up pretty easily. If you train your child to use an escape hood, make a big impression that they cannot put anything else over their head, like plastic bags or other dangerous things.
- If you are ever directly exposed to a nerve agent, you will only have seconds to respond. Move as quickly as you can from the area and call for help. EMTs carry a drug called Atropine that can counteract the affects of many different types of nerve agent. Small devices called auto-injectors can be used to inject measured amounts of Atropine that can help to reduce the agent's deadly effects.

   At this time, auto-injector kits are only available to professional responders, the military and other qualified personnel. If you are a frequent subway rider and have first aid or emergency medical training, you might want to consider carrying auto-injector kits when you ride the subway. Atropine auto-injector kits are not sold to the general public, but only to EMTs, firefighters, police and other first responders.

There are two more reasonable precautions to make your subway ride safer. The first is to wear a half-face medical respirator (3M P-95) like the ones worn by Japanese subway passengers, or even like the ones described in the emergency transportation chapter. They will provide you with a small amount of protection from some chemical and bio agents.

CHAPTER 17

Fire Prevention
and Escape

THE BEST PREPAREDNESS FOR FIRES—AN EMERGENCY ALL TOO FREQUENTLY ENCOUNTERED—
is prevention. This chapter will teach you how to take measures in your home, apartment, and workplace to reduce the risk of fires starting, and how to escape them if they do.

Fire Safety for the Home

- Install smoke detectors and carbon monoxide detectors in your home.
- Check smoke detectors every six months, and change batteries once a year.
- Never leave or burn candles near curtains, drapes, or other flammable fabric.
- All combustible materials (paint thinner, canned insect spray, lighter fluid, and so on) should be stored in a safe location away from heat, flame, or sources of electrical sparks.
- Garbage must be removed regularly, never allowed to accumulate. Do not place trash near stoves, electrical outlets, or any other sources of electrical sparks or flames.

Electrical Equipment Safeguards

- Do not plug extension or adapter cords into other adapter cords, and never run cords under carpets. Eventually, the insulation will be worn away by foot traffic and the exposed wire can cause a short circuit and ignite the carpet.
- High-current devices like office machines, microwave ovens, toasters or television sets should have their own sockets. Never group more than one high-current appliance together in one outlet.
- Do not place flammable things near electrical outlets where they could rub against or fall onto the plug and cause a short circuit and fire.
- Unplug all idle electrical devices.
- Replace all burned-out fuses.

- Place extra smoke escape hoods in easy-to-reach locations around your home.
- Use only UL-approved electrical devices. Frayed wires, defective appliances, and other potential electrical fire hazards must be repaired or replaced.

Fire Safeguards for the Kitchen

- Keep an ABC fire extinguisher in or near your kitchen.
- Keep your stove clean and grease free.
- Take extra care when cooking with oil.
- Do not leave your stove on and unattended.
- Periodically check the pilots on your gas stovetop to make sure they are lit and clean.
- If a fire in your apartment is too big to put out with an extinguisher, gather your family and Grab-and-Go Bags and quickly evacuate. If you can't grab the bag within ten seconds, leave it behind. Every second that you hesitate increases your chances of being trapped inside, especially if you live in an old building. Close the door (but leave it unlocked), and alert your neighbors as you leave.
- If the fire produces heavy smoke and you have a smoke escape hood, put it on before you leave your apartment.
- Do not use elevators to evacuate. Move out through the closest stairwell. If the stairwell is too crowded, quickly seek another exit route such as a fire escape, other emergency exit, or less crowded stairwell.
- Do not open doors that feel hot.
- If you have a disabled or elderly neighbor, help him or her out of the building.
- If you have young children, never leave them unsupervised. It takes only a few minutes to perish from a fire. Nothing is worth the risk leaving them alone.
- If you have children, keep all lighters, matches, candles and all flammable materials hidden and out of their reach.
- If you are trapped inside and can get to a window, hang a blanket or towel out of the window. Firemen who see it will try to help you.
- If it becomes too dangerous to stay near a window, find a safer location and take a pan or other noisemaker to help rescuers find you. If gasoline vapor or natural gas is present, strike a non-sparking surface with a non-metallic object.
- Wet a towel and place it under a door to block smoke until help arrives.

- Move flammable things away from exits, including curtains, garbage, and any other stuff that could ignite and block your path with flames.
- If you have window gates, keep your keys near the window for quick emergency use.
- If you live in a building with a terrace and are below the fire, move outside and wait for help.

Fire Safety Tips for Smokers

If you smoke, your household is nearly twice as likely to have a fire as a non-smoker's. If you have a drinking or other substance abuse problem, the risk goes up even more. Cigarette tobacco is treated with chemicals to keep it lit. A snuffed cigarette may seem unlit, but tiny sparks that linger inside are not visible...Cigarette smokers should be mindful of where they dispose of their butts. Never put a tobacco or marijuana cigarette or cigar in the trash.

- Never smoke in bed.
- Ashtrays should be heavy and made of glass or metal.
- Never leave a lit cigarette, cigar, or pipe on a table or cabinet edge. As the cigarette burns, its balance shifts, and it can fall to the floor and ignite a carpet or any flammable material.

If you smoke cigarettes, the best fire safety improvement is to find the willpower to give up the habit. If you don't, observe the measures above to protect yourself and your loved ones from cigarette fires. If you have a favorite recliner in which you like to smoke and drink, coat it in Flameguard 80, Pyrogard SRF, or some other flame retardant. You may want to consider saturating your mattress and bedclothes in flame retardant as well.

High-Rise Fire Escape

High-rise structural fires are dangerous, as their height and layout make firefighting and emergency rescue difficult. Most modern high-rise buildings are designed to contain fires in one area, but they are not made to suppress the toxic smoke that can fill a building in minutes. If you live or work in a high-rise building, you need a detailed survival and escape plan.

- Learn the locations of every exit. Check to see if they are locked or have obstructions that would block or slow your evacuation. If you find a locked emergency exit or stairway, notify the landlord or building manager. By law, they must see to it that all emergency exits are clear. If your building does not conduct regular fire drills, encourage them to do so.
- Report hazardous conditions in your building to the local fire and sanitation department and continue to complain until the problem is solved.

Acquire the protective equipment that will help you escape from a fire. Generally, the best choice during a high-rise building fire is to stay put and wait for help. But if you are not a safe distance from the fire, you will need to escape the heat and concentrated smoke. Your equipment will help you survive the smoke and navigate your exit. The most important fire escape items to have in high-rise apartments or offices are smoke escape hoods and high-power, non-incendive flashlights. Every employee and resident should have their own smoke escape hood and flashlight.

Fire blankets provide a temporary barrier against flame and heat, and each person in your home or office should have one (preferably the water gel-coated kind favored by stuntmen).

Technon, the company that manufactures the Breath of Life emergency escape mask, has also created the Firefly survival poncho, a fire-resistant, aluminized fiberglass coverall. During a fire, you may be forced to move through an area where you are exposed to high temperatures or flames. The Firefly can protect you for short periods from heat up to 1,650° F.

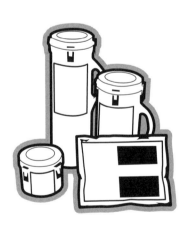

Various Water-Jel Fire Blankets

They are easy to slip on and can give you the ability to quickly move through a fire without sustaining serious life-threatening burns. It comes in a small briefcase that can be placed in your bedroom, home, or work area. It comes in sizes that fit adults and children.

Emergency escape ladders are useful, because high-rise fires rarely engulf entire floors or burn more than three stories at a time. If you are caught in the burning area, emergency escape ladders let you climb below the fire to a safer area.

Successful use of these ladders requires regular drills and, in group settings, selection of ladder captains responsible for setup and deployment. Captains should be physically fit and unafraid of heights; their duties will be installing the ladder rapidly and correctly, climbing down below the fire line, breaking a window, and serving as the anchor to help the other evacuees.

All high-rise buildings should be equipped with emergency light systems that switch on during fires and power outages, illuminating staircases and hallways.

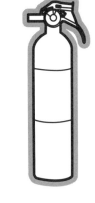

ABC Fire Extinguisher

- High-rise elevators should be equipped with pry bars to open jammed doors and insulated work gloves to prevent electrical shock in case the pry bar touches a live line.
- A large pry bar (at least 36"), claw tool, and axe should be mounted near the exit and near an emergency light fixture.
- A powerful rechargeable emergency spotlight should be placed near each exit.
- An ABC fire extinguisher should be placed at every entrance and exit and in any area with lots of combustible material. A Water-Jel fire blanket should also be included in an area that is easy to reach.
- A comprehensive first aid kit must be placed in an accessible area in your office, and at least one out of ten of your workers should be trained in emergency first aid.

Extreme Fire Escape Methods

In a worst case scenario, emergency smoke escape hoods, ladders, and high-powered flashlights may not be enough. If you are strong and physically fit, you might consider rappelling, which is my personal high-rise fire escape method of choice.

Those interested in learning to rappel for escape—and mountaineering—should be able to find a school or sports center nearby for professional instruction. Books and videos with useful information about rappelling and necessary gear are widely available.

Once you have learned the techniques, you can assemble your own rappelling kit or get a pre-packaged emergency escape kit like the one sold by Life Safety Equipment, which has 60 feet of rope—enough to descend six stories. Buying your own rope lets you go even further.

Acquiring rappelling and ascending skills and a small emergency kit will provide you with reliable methods to escape from high-rise fires and structural failures. Some emergency rescue system packages are especially designed for the physically challenged and injured. If you have disabled family members or co-workers, help them develop an escape plan. With the proper training and specialized equipment, you will be able to help disabled persons escape from harm.

In some extreme cases, such as an attack similar to the destruction of the World Trade Center, rappelling or ascending gear may not be helpful. If you ever find yourself in this type of situation, your final option is an emergency escape parachute. This is a risky last-chance measure, but parachutes designed for emergency escape from high-rise buildings are available, *e.g.,* Aerial Egress' High Office Parachute Escape (HOPE), designed for those with no skydiving experience.

The HOPE system uses a WWII-style round parachute. Systems that include rectangular, maneuverable, glider-style parachutes put novice users at a higher risk of losing control and corkscrewing too fast to the street.

Fires are not only one of the most frequently encountered emergencies, they are also the most terrifying. I have been in two major house fires in my lifetime and that is two too many. To survive fires it's important to conduct drills to make your response to a fire reflexive. With fires, he who hesitates is lost. No matter how strong and fast you think you may be, the smoke is stronger and the fire is faster.

Teach your children what to do and practice with them. It helps to build their confidence and sense of independence and may give them that extra edge they need to keep alive and uninjured.

This chapter is dedicated to the memory of Justina Braithwaite and her brother Justin, two children who died in a fire that was suspiciously set at their Brooklyn home in 2003. Their hardworking mother made a tragic mistake and left Justina and Justin home alone to work a night shift. Little Justina, age nine, who suffered from sickle cell anemia, struggled valiantly to try and save her one-year-old brother from the flames. They died together.

CHAPTER 18

Extreme Weather

Category 1
Sustained wind speed 74–95 mph
Storm surge 4–5 feet
Minimal damage. Downed power and communication lines, street signs, unanchored mobile homes, trees and other forms of vegetation.

Category 2
Sustained wind speed 96–110 mph
Storm surge 6–8 feet
Moderate damage. Overturned mobile homes, small boats capsized, flash flooding, torn rooftops, communication and power lines knocked down.

Category 3
Sustained wind speed 111–130 mph
Storm surge 9–12 feet
Extensive damage. Small wooden structures may be destroyed. Many small steel-reinforced concrete structures (gas stations) can be severely damaged. Roads will be blocked by fallen debris. Live power lines will be exposed.

Category 4
Sustained wind speed 131–155 mph
Storm surge 13–18 feet
Extreme damage. Homes will be destroyed, steel reinforced concrete buildings will sustain heavy superficial damage, roads will be cut off, homes flooded.

Category 5
Sustained wind speed 155–175 mph
Storm surge 18–25 feet
Catastrophic damage.

METEOROLOGISTS ARE BEGINNING TO IDENTIFY LINKS BETWEEN GLOBAL WARMING AND THE increasing power of tropical storms, said the respected journal *Science* in September 2005.

The number of severe hurricanes has increased by 80 percent over the past 35 years. Rising temperatures are beginning to melt glaciers and polar ice sheets.

By the year 2100, our climate will warm by one degree overall, and the seas will rise four inches, projects the National Center for Atmospheric Research (NCAR). Other studies say the situation is much worse, and that by 2100 the global temperature will rise over six degrees and the sea level will rise by more than a foot. These conditions will flood coastal regions, erode away islands and further increase the ferocity of hurricanes, tornadoes and even winter storms. Enormous heat waves and droughts will damage agriculture globally and exacerbate fresh water supply problems. The spread of disease is also an expected result of global warming.

To develop the proper preparedness, response, and recovery strategies for extreme weather emergencies, you must first determine what you might encounter. Here are The Unlucky Seven, and guidance on how to survive them best:

Hurricanes

Hurricanes strike all areas along the American East Coast, the Gulf of Mexico and the Caribbean. Hurricanes also spawn large tropical storms (microbursts and tornadoes) with torrential rainfall that triggers extensive flooding and mudslides in the southwest United States, Mexico, and occasionally the Pacific Coast. As we have seen in New Orleans, Mississippi, Alabama and Texas, hurricanes can produce catastrophic damage to coastal cities, towns and even communities hundreds of miles away from the storm center.

A hurricane's power is measured by its destructive potential, wind speed, and central pressure. They are broken up into five different categories on what is called the Saffir-Simpson Hurricane Scale.

We can expect to encounter many more powerful storms over the course of the next few decades. Anyone who lives in, or in hundred-mile proximity to "hurricane alley" should prepare a hurricane escape plan with all of your family members and rehearse it during hurricane season. Make a detailed list of all of your needs that includes:

- Your evacuation destination.
- Mode of transportation.
- Number of family members in tow.
- Critical items to take.
- Amount of money needed to evacuate.
- Prescription medicines (if needed).
- Location of hotels, area hospitals at point of evacuation.
- Gas stations along route and extra emergency supplies for auto (if driving).
- Personal protection.
- Transport cage if you have a pet.
- Food, water, portable toilet with odor-absorbing cat litter, hand-crank radio and some entertainment (music, cards, games).
- Make sure that all of your gutters and downspouts are clear.
- If you have the time to do so, you might want to consider creating an emergency cache of precious items that you want to protect but don't or can't take with you. You can place family heirlooms and other must-keep items inside this storage canister to store away in the safety of your own backyard. If your home is destroyed by a hurricane, your precious items will be safely tucked away underground. Fifty-five-gallon steel or plastic drums with removable lids are great for cacheing. Wrap each individual item in plastic trash bags (if the item is made of metal, you will need to coat it with oil to prevent corrosion). Seal them up tightly without puncturing the bags, making certain that it is an airtight seal, and carefully place the item(s) inside the barrel. Once the barrel is full, stretch another plastic bag like a membrane over the top. This will serve as an O-ring seal to minimize moisture from entering the barrel while it is buried. Make certain not to bury it near a septic tank, power lines or water pipes. You should also do it under the cover of darkness so that no one else can see where you have placed your buried treasure.
- Purchase strong storm shutters and have them placed on your windows. You should also use marine plywood sheets ⅝" custom cut to fit your windows.
- If you live near large trees, cut off any loose branches.

- If you live on high ground, it would also be a good idea to build an emergency shelter (also see tornado section in this chapter).

If You Are Not Able to Evacuate and Must Ride Out the Hurricane, Take the Following Precautionary Measures:

- Move all outdoor furniture or any other loose objects on your property inside your home.
- Close all outside and interior doors, storm shutters and windows. Shut your gas at the main valve and turn off all your propane tanks (if you have them). Disconnect non-essential appliances. Turn your refrigerator up to its highest level and do not open the doors until after the storm passes. This will help preserve your refrigerated food supply during any possible blackouts.
- If you do not have an emergency supply of water stored away in your home, fill up every pot, bottle and even your bathtub with water (clean the tub first).
- As the storm nears your home, stay away from windows. Put on a helmet (doesn't have to be a hard hat, could be a bicycle helmet) to protect your head from falling debris. Keep your Grab-and-Go Bag within sight. Have your raincoat handy and be prepared to leave your home and find shelter if you must. If you have small children, prepare to tether them to you with a good thick cord. Keep your multi-tool or a sharp knife handy. Evacuation during a hurricane is a dangerous option that should only be made as a last resort.
- Keep your radio on to stay on top of important information.
- If you have a workbench or sturdy four-legged table in your home you can lie underneath. You can also use your bathtub as a shield.
- You can also take refuge in a small closet, or, if it's safe from flooding, a corner in your basement. Try and stay in the corner nearest to the direction of the wind.
- If you live in a mobile home or trailer near a coastline, river, or creek, it is best to evacuate to a Red Cross designated shelter before the hurricane hits.
- After the hurricane passes, wait until daylight to assess the damage. Beware of sharp debris, fallen live power lines, holes, weakened floors, staircases and other hazards. If you have a working cellphone, limit calls to the early morning or evening when the traffic is lower. Look out for frightened stray dogs and agitated homeowners who may mistake you for a looter.

- If necessary, locate an area in your neighborhood that you can use as a temporary shelter until help arrives. Make sure to bring water, food and other supplies. Keep yourself hydrated, and avoid walking through floodwaters.

Severe Thunderstorms

A thunderstorm is classified as severe if it produces hail, wind of 58+ mph and/or flash floods. Dangerous storms can produce large hailstones, mudslides from torrential rain, flash flooding, and in some cases, small tornadoes (F-0 to F-1 on the Fujita scale). Three hundred people are injured and 80 people are killed by lightning strikes in the United States every year. In the western states, electrical storms spark wildfires that destroy wildlife and hundreds of homes, and create billions of dollars of property damage annually.

The most severe thunderstorms can linger for long periods of time. Thunderstorms can also appear in clusters; as one moves away, another moves in. Most produce heavy rains from 15 minutes to one hour. The most severe variety develop in hot and humid conditions in the late spring, summer and fall.

Flooding and communications failures and power outages are caused by lightning strikes and fallen trees. They can also cause minor transportation disruptions, property damage, and severe or fatal injuries.

When you see inclement weather approaching, tune in to the NOAA weather radio station, or your local radio or TV news programs for information. Doppler systems can actually pinpoint areas where lightning strikes. Many local weather reports now issue severe thunderstorm warnings that you can use to prepare and protect yourself from harm.

When Encountering Thunderstorms:

- Seek shelter. If you are outdoors, quickly discontinue your activities and find an area that can provide you with safe cover (not trees). Buildings, underpasses, tunnels, caves are the best areas; a hard-top car can be used in a pinch even though this cannot be considered entirely safe because if it struck by lightning, you might be injured. But taking shelter in a car is far preferable than staying in the open. When sitting inside a car, make sure to keep your hands off of metal objects.
- If you are in a forest, find shelter in a low-lying area under a heavy growth of small trees. In an open area, search for the lowest area you can find. If you feel your hair standing on end, a lightning bolt is about

to strike. Quickly squat down low, balancing your body weight on the balls of your feet. Cover your ears and place your head between your knees. Make yourself as small a target as possible and minimize your contact with the ground. If you lie flat you will not only increase your target size but expose yourself to more electrical energy if a lightning bolt strikes nearby.

■ Always follow the 30/30 lighting safety rule. This means you should seek shelter if thunder comes before you count to 30 after seeing a lightning strike. You should stay indoors for at least 30 minutes after hearing the last thunderclap.

■ If you are riding a bicycle or motorcycle or you're standing near any vehicle and a storm is rapidly approaching, take cover quickly and stand away from your bike. The metal attracts lightning. If you are on a golf course, move away from the clubs and find shelter. Those giant golf umbrellas tend to become fancy lightning rods during a thunderstorm—leave them behind.

■ If you are on a beach and hear a thunderstorm approaching, give yourself plenty of time to find shelter. Beaches are dangerous places during electrical storms. So are open fields, boats, outhouses and other similar small structures.

■ If you are indoors and using a computer, unplug it along with other appliances, including your television. Thunderstorms produce power surges that can do serious damage to your equipment. It is a common myth that surge protectors will protect against damage from a lightning strike. They don't.

■ If you live in a small home, wait until the storm passes to shower or bathe. Your plumbing can conduct dangerous electrical charges created by lightning.

If You Are With Someone Who is Struck by Lightning:

■ Check for a strong pulse. If it is present, examine for burns or trauma caused by falling.

■ If the person is conscious, check if there is a loss of hearing or eyesight. This must be reported to EMTs or paramedics.

■ If breathing has stopped, and if you know how to administer mouth-to-mouth resuscitation, do it until help arrives.

■ If the heart has stopped and you know CPR, administer it until help arrives.

Floods

In the Northeast, flooding is often created by cyclonic storm fronts called *Nor'easters* that can produce heavy rain, snow and turbulent tidal conditions that cause erosion of coastal areas and heavy flooding. In the South, flooding is primarily caused by hurricanes and severe rainstorms. All 50 states experience some kind of severe flooding.

Flooding can disrupt transportation, power and communication, and cause water pumping, filtration and sewage treatment problems. Floods can be limited to small areas, or spread out hundreds of square miles from river basins. The types of floods vary, but the most dangerous can be flash floods, which occur after torrential rainfall, or dam breaks. Powerful rushing waters can easily sweep away everything in their path including automobiles and homes. Floodwaters can also be filled with dangerous debris such as rocks, shards of glass, metal and mud. Rainfall or a storm surge can also cause a river to overflow its banks, as seen in New Orleans during the Katrina disaster, where levees failed to hold back overland flooding, causing flash flood-like conditions. Floods can occur anywhere, but people who live in low-lying areas near rivers, lakes, dams, the ocean, or any reasonably-sized body of water including reservoirs and dried-up lakebeds, are advised to make special preparations.

If You Live in an Area Prone to Flooding:

- Homeowners are advised to purchase flood insurance.
- Don't move to a floodplain. The local office of emergency management should have floodplain maps available that can help you choose a safe homesite. If you must build in this type of area, make certain to build a reinforced foundation or elevate your home above projected flood water levels.
- If you plan to build a home in an area prone to flooding, consider a geodesic dome. They are more flood-resistant than the usual home and easy enough to clean off in case of inundation by water.
- Build barriers around your home such as water channels, small levees and floodwalls that can redirect the path of floodwaters away from your home.
- If you have a basement, use sealant and waterproofing compounds (PVC) on the walls to prevent or reduce absorption. Every crack is a potential leak point. If floodwater is absorbed into your basement walls, you run the risk of developing dangerous mold that can produce neuro-

logical and immunological damage. Most of the homes in New Orleans will need to be completely destroyed because of mold.

■ The electrical junction box, furnace, and water heater should be raised as high as possible. Keep precious items stored in the highest point of your home. Family photos should be copied, and the originals placed in airtight bags containing desiccants to absorb surrounding moisture.

■ To prevent floodwater from backing up into your storm drains, install devices called check valves.

■ If you have small children, or a sick or elderly family member in your home, invest in an inflatable raft or small boat that can be pulled through floodwaters. If you can't afford one, you will need to find a large and buoyant enough float. Large wooden tabletops, inflatable mattresses, and other decent-size floatable objects can be used as emergency boats. For the kids and babies, an inflated tire or a kiddie pool will work but you cannot allow the children to carry sharp toys. You will also need to keep an eye out for sharp debris. Tie a strong line around the child's waist; make certain to double up their shirts to prevent rope burn and loosely wrap the line around your upper body, so as not to drag the child under in case you fall. Fasten the end of the line tightly around the neck of a two-liter soda bottle with the cap tightly screwed on: if the line is dropped in the water, this will keep it floating and easy to find.

■ Purchase a hand-crank shortwave radio or scanner and tune into the NOAA weather radio channel. You can also check with local TV and radio stations. All should give you advance warning about potential floods. If you receive information that indicates a large flood is possible, gather up money, toiletries, critical documents, prescription medicine, ID, birth certificate, insurance, deed, will, etc. Seal them up in watertight plastic bags with the desiccants, pack them into your E-Kit or Grab-and-Go Bags, and immediately make your way to a shelter in an area with higher ground. If you're warned of a flash flood, quickly grab what you can and immediately move to higher ground on foot. Check on elderly neighbors who may need your assistance and gather a group of able-bodied folk who can help to move them to safety.

■ If you live near a river, stream, drainage ditch, reservoir, canyon, dry lake bed or any other flood-prone areas, remember that flash floods can suddenly occur without warning.

■ Purchase a pair of wading pants or irrigation boots for every member of the family. They can be expensive, but if you ever find yourself slogging through filthy floodwaters you will be glad you acquired them. You should also have a walking stick handy to help keep your balance and move floating objects out of the way.

If You Must Evacuate Your Home:

- Secure your home. If you have time, bring in outdoor furniture. Move essential items to an upper floor.
- Disconnect all electrical appliances, TV and tools. Turn off your electrical power at the junction box and your gas at the main valve. Don't attempt to shut down any electrical devices if you are wet or standing in floodwater.
- Tighten all the gas caps on your vehicles and heating fuel tanks to minimize seepage if they are submerged.
- Place your Grab-and-Go Bag inside three large heavy-duty trash bags. Capture extra air inside the bag by opening them wide before sealing them up. Tie the bags tightly at the top to form an airtight seal. Wrap a strong thick cord around the knot at the top and tie a tether line to your waist. The bag should float, and you can drag it through the waters behind you.
- Never drive into an area that has been flooded. Floodwaters can be deceptively deep. If you drive into an area with water over two feet deep, you will need to abandon your vehicle and step into dangerous floodwaters. All it takes is six to eight inches of water to stall out most cars.
- Don't try to walk through moving water. Rushing water that is only ankle-deep can easily knock you off your feet. Carry your walking stick and poke the ground, checking for holes or weak spots as you walk.
- If you live in the South, watch for dangerous reptiles such as water moccasins, coral snakes and alligators.
- Wear swimmers' goggles to protect your eyes from filthy water.
- Beware of spots near fallen or buried power lines. This water may be electrically charged and can electrocute you or cause serious burns.
- Avoid moving through floodwaters because they are almost always contaminated with sewage and toxic chemicals. If you live in proximity to a chemical plant, fuel storage or waste processing facility, you can expect that the floodwaters contain a mix of everything they process or store. If you have open sores, cuts or bruises on your lower extremities, you're at risk at developing infections. As a result of Katrina, people in the New Orleans area were infected with *Vibrio vulnificus,* a flesh-eating water-borne organism closely related to the bacterium that causes cholera. Avoid getting floodwater into your mouth, eyes, ears or nose.
- Do not enter flooded buildings; there may be flood-created structural weaknesses that can cause a collapse.

- Don't drive on areas where floodwaters have receded. Supporting dirt and gravel may have eroded away, and the weight of an automobile or truck could trigger a collapse.
- If you cannot swim, do not attempt to move through floodwaters unless you can find something to use as a flotation device. A group of empty two-liter soda bottles with caps fastened tightly and stuffed into a heavy-duty trash bag can do the trick. Fasten yourself to the improvised flotation device with wire, twine or any other cord that you can find. If you cannot improvise a flotation device, climb to the highest point you can find and still be visible with your gear bag, a white towel and broom, and wait for assistance. In your E-Kit you should have a whistle to signal for help.

After the Flood

After you return home, you will need to clean everything that was exposed to the toxic floodwaters. See Chapter 6 for its discussion of Personal Protective Equipment. This should include your partial face respirator (R-100, 95 class) and a non-permeable coverall with hood, goggles and a broad-spectrum industrial-strength disinfectant like Encore needed to kill fungi, viruses, and other virulent microorganisms. Do not attempt to wash away mud or any residue without respiratory protection unless you want toxic material to take up residence inside your lungs.

- If your dog or cat is exposed to the toxic floodwaters, they will need to be thoroughly cleaned with strong animal shampoo.
- Don't drink any tap water in your area until long after the floodwater has receded. Many of the chemicals and bacteria in the floodwaters will linger in the soil long after the water has dried. Minute quantities of these organisms and substances can seep into water pipes through microscopic cracks. Some organisms like cryptosporidium are resistant to the extra chlorine that filtration plants add after flooding. If you must drink tap water, try to boil it first, and purchase a filter at your local supermarket such as the types made by Brita, or PUR.

Tornadoes

A tornado is a whirling juggernaut of a storm that can completely destroy all but the most sturdily built steel-reinforced concrete structures in its path. The Fujita scale is used to gauge the power of a tornado by assessing the damage it produces after it passes over a structure. F-0 is the lowest rating, F-5 the highest with wind speeds in excess of 300 mph.

Tornadoes vary in appearance. Some have the telltale funnel cloud while others are not as apparent. On some occasions, tornadoes may develop without warning and the wind may become very calm. In fact, the skies may appear clear and sunny.

To Prepare for Tornadoes:

- Keeping an eye out for approaching thunderstorms. Watch for dark low clouds, torrential rains, and large hailstones followed by loud roaring sounds. These conditions can sometimes mark the development of tornadoes. Monitor the NOAA weather channel or local radio and TV programs to check for tornado warnings. If you are under a tornado warning you must immediately find a storm cellar or a building constructed from steel-reinforced concrete.
- If you are caught outside when a tornado develops and cannot find shelter nearby, lie flat in a low-lying area or ditch. Cover your head with your hands. Stay alert! Flash flooding can also occur during tornadoes. If you are in a non-steel-reinforced concrete structure, move toward the center. Find a strong non-glass table and get under it. Use your hands to protect your head and neck. Most injuries and fatalities are caused by flying debris. Don't seek out underpasses unless they are very strong. If you find one, move toward the corner farthest away from the approaching tornado and lay down flat.
- Trailers or mobile homes are dangerous places when a tornado strikes. Immediately escape to a nearby storm shelter or strong building.

If you live in a tornado-prone region, and have construction experience, consider building a "safe room" in your house. This is a special area reinforced with concrete and steel designed to resist the winds and flying debris created by tornadoes. Even better, you can purchase a readymade storm shelter. They are safer than homemade safe rooms and can withstand the worst storms and floods. Check the Preparedness Source List Chapter for further information on storm shelters.

Winter Storms

(Blizzards, Freezing Rain, Extreme Cold)

If you live in a northern region, you know how dangerous large winter storms can be. Many are so severe that they can shut down air and ground transportation and cause communications disruptions, power outages, flooding and heating problems. Blocked roads can cause disruptions in medical services and food, gas and heating oil deliveries.

Hypothermia may strike the less fortunate victims of winter storms. The weight of snow can sometimes cause rooftops to cave in at homes and even shopping malls. Automobile accidents are common because of visibility problems and ice sheets that cover roads. Extreme cold can rupture water mains, cutting off running water. This is a major problem for firefighters who need access to water from fire hydrants. You should have a solid plan in place to deal with contingencies caused by winter storms. Begin by keeping the following equipment handy.

- Wide shovel/snow blower.
- Rock salt—to prevent the formation of ice on driveways and walkways.
- Sand—for traction if your vehicle is stuck in a snowbank or ice.
- Blowtorch—for frozen locks.
- Small pike—to chop away ice.

Make sure you have enough supplies in your home to ride out a severe storm. A large blizzard or extreme cold spell may force you to stay indoors for long periods of time; consider having enough to sustain you until the emergency passes.

Prepare a checklist that includes all of the items that you and your family need to hunker down for a two-week minimum. This would include non-perishable food, fuel (for your vehicles and heating), firewood (if you own a fireplace), extra fuel canisters for gas-powered space heaters, batteries, extra medications (if you are a prescription drug user), water, soap, and any other material that you would consider to be critical—even some not-so-critical items such as DVDs and CDs to help break up the monotony of being homebound.

Make sure that your home or apartment is "winterized." This can be accomplished by weather-stripping all of your doors and windows or installing efficient storm windows. Caulking all cracks and gaps will also help to reduce heat loss. Insulate your walls, attics, air conditioning vents and as a last-resort measure, cover your windows with plastic garbage bags. Stretch them tightly across the window and duct-tape them down. Not only will they help to insulate, they can also function as low-grade solar heaters if your home or apartment is exposed to direct sunlight.

Winterize Your Vehicle:

- Keep your car or truck filled with antifreeze.
- Keep your gas tank full.
- The battery should be fully charged, and the ignition in good working order. If battery terminals are corroded, they should be cleaned.
- Your window defroster, thermostat, and heater, must be fully functional along with the windshield wipers.
- All lights should be in working order.
- Brakes should be inspected by a mechanic before the winter season.
- Snow tires are must-have items. The studded type are best, especially if you are a commuter that must drive in hazardous conditions. You should also own tire chains.
- Your exhaust system must also be inspected by a mechanic. Carbon monoxide leaks during the winter months are an extreme hazard because windows are usually shut.
- Purchase a portable power supply (jump-starter) just in case your battery goes dead. It is difficult to find someone to jump-start your car in a blizzard. Certain units can also provide power for tools and other electrical devices.
- Replace your oil. 5–30 grade is best for winter driving.
- Replace all air and fuel filters.
- Use a moisture removal additive in your fuel to prevent frozen fuel lines.
- Add "ballast" to increase road traction of your vehicle. This can be accomplished by placing some sandbags or concrete blocks in the trunk and under your seats to give the car added weight.
- Keep your car's Grab-and-Go Bag handy at all times, and make sure it has blankets, candles, water, road flares, a small shovel and ice pick.

If You're Trapped in a Car During a Blizzard:

- Drive off to the side of a main road or highway. Turn on your hazard lights. Find a piece of cloth to hang on your antenna or a stick to improvise a distress flag. If you have a road flare, you would need to find a spot where it could burn without sinking into the snow.
- Stay in your car. If you are near a main road or highway, you will eventually be found by rescuers or snow plow teams. Don't try to walk unless

you are close to a building that you know is unlocked and heated and can be used for shelter.

- Turn on your engine to run the heater for about 20 minutes each hour to keep warm. Anything less than 20 minutes may risk the engine becoming too cold to start up again. While it is running, crack a window to maintain some fresh air circulation. Every hour, clear snow from the exhaust pipe to prevent carbon monoxide from backing up into the vehicle.
- To maintain body heat, use road maps, seat covers, floor mats and if you aren't alone, other passengers, to keep yourself warm. Drape your coat over your body like a blanket. If you have an infant with you, button or zip them up inside your clothing allowing their bodies to make direct skin contact.
- Drink fluids.
- Stay alert! You must be prepared to flag down rescue crews if they appear nearby. If you have another passenger, take turns resting.
- Don't burn out your battery by keeping the radio on. Always carry a hand-crank radio in your vehicle.
- In the night, keep your windows clear of snow and your flashlight or indoor light on so rescuers can see you.
- If you are in a remote area, you will need to take more drastic measures to attract attention. Every hour or so, you will need to dig out a distress signal in the snow—SOS is best. You will need to repeat this frequently because the heavy snow will cover it up quickly. Line the signal with tree limbs, rocks or garbage to attract the attention of rescuers. Include an arrow that points in the direction where you vehicle is stuck.
- If you have a kerosene heater in your kit, make sure to keep it away from anything flammable inside the vehicle and keep the window cracked for ventilation.
- Wait until the blizzard is over before you move out on foot to seek assistance.

One of the most common physical dangers of winter storms is overexertion. Many people shoveling snow from driveways and digging out buried cars suffer from heart attacks. If you are not in good health, you may even want to invest in a snow blower.

Frostbite is also another common cold weather injury. If you lose feeling in your toes, fingers, ears, nose or any other extremity, you need to seek out medical assistance. Hypothermia, another dangerous cold-weather physical emergency, has the following symptoms: uncontrollable shivering, disorientation, slurred speech, extreme fatigue, drowsiness, incoherence and memory loss. People suffering from hypothermia should be moved to a warm area, have their wet clothing removed, and warm wet cloths used to heat the center of the body. Give them warm non-alcoholic beverages and get them some medical attention as quickly as possible.

Drought and Heat Waves

Back in August 2003, Europe suffered through a massive heat wave that claimed an estimated 35,000 lives. Atmospheric warming can increase the number and severity of droughts, and we will almost certainly experience more similar situations.

Heat exhaustion is a mild form of shock brought about by the redirection of blood flow to the skin from vital organs. Without medical treatment, the body's temperature will continue to rise until heat stroke and death occurs. Heatstroke is when your body's temperature regulation system shuts down. Without it, your body temperature rises quickly to levels that produce permanent brain damage and death if left untreated.

Heat waves also cause power outages, water and air quality problems, transportation delays. We must prepare for such future events as:

- Water Shortages: Desert states such as New Mexico, Arizona, Nevada, Utah, California, and parts of Colorado may soon experience freshwater shortages that will reach critical levels.
- Forest Fires: Reduced rainfall will convert many forest areas into dry tinder.
- Diseases: Lack of rainfall in desert states will aid the spread of diseases such as Hantavirus.
- Loss of Agriculture: Small and large farms will be destroyed by droughts.
- Economic downturn: Jobs in the agriculture industry will be lost.

Droughts are difficult events to prepare for because they require the ability to store away huge amounts of water. Large fresh water tanks can be purchased by some homeowners and buried in their backyards, but this is still only a short-term solution for a long-term problem.

The best methods of drought and heat wave preparedness involve conservation and common sense practical methods.

- Retrofit your home's plumbing fixtures with water conserving devices. This includes installing low-flow showerheads, toilets, and even low water use dishwashers that can save thousands of gallons of water per year.

- Maintain a larger emergency water supply in a large water tank (for drinking and firefighting purposes). You may also need a small gas-powered high-pressure water pump and extra water hoses.
- If you live in an area near large amounts of vegetation, develop a solid response-and-escape protocol in case of fire.
- If you live in a wood structure, you should consider having your roof coated with a substance called sodium silicate. When added to wood and exposed to flame, it will not support combustion. Sodium silicate also repels termites.
- If your home is near overhanging tree branches, consider cutting them down for safety purposes.

IA TIP

If you are a diabetic, you may want to consider purchasing a small battery- or solar- powered refrigerator. During power outages, you may need a method to keep your insulin refrigerated. Sun Frost manufactures the RFVB vaccine refrigerator freezer, designed to accommodate medication that needs to be cooled. They also make other small refrigerators that you can use to keep cold drinks handy if the power goes down.

- Always keep your freezers filled with ice. If the power goes down, the ice will help to keep frozen foods fresh. Keep in mind that freezers and refrigerators are essentially giant thermoses designed to keep the cold air inside from escaping. Open the refrigerator door only when you need to.
- If you don't have an air conditioner, keep your windows open at all times while you are at home. If you live in an apartment you might need to install a security gate to protect your home from potential burglars.
- Reduce clutter. The cleaner your home is, the easier it is to cool off. Piles of loose clothing and papers function like heat sinks helping to keep the temperature in your home or apartment high.

Mudslides

Mudslides can happen anywhere and can produce tremendous amounts of property damage and death. In October 1988, Hurricane Mitch triggered mudslides in Honduras that killed over 7000 people. More recently, many were killed by slides in the Dominican Republic, Philippines, Haiti and even Southern California in Spring, 2005.

With severe storms on the rise, we should be concerned about the increasing frequency and magnitude of mudslides, and must begin to develop preparedness protocols that will allow us to escape their most destructive effects.

- Never build or buy a home built near a mountain edge, slope, drainage way or at the top or middle of a valley.
- Watch for changes in the shape of your surrounding landscape after heavy rainfall. Check for leaning street signs, fences, utility poles, trees or dimpled patches in the ground, or warped center or dividing lines in the road.
- If you notice in your home that windows and doors are beginning to stick, shifting soil may have caused movement in your home's foundation. Check for developing cracks in your walkway and misaligned staircases.

Watch Out for Mudslides If:

- Rumbling and cracking sounds get progressively louder.
- Ground shifts.
- Automobile alarms go off. Many will be triggered by the shifting ground.
- Restless animals; dogs may begin to bark and birds chirp loudly as they do before earthquakes.
- Water pipes may be ruptured by the shifting earth and you may spot water bubbling up to the surface. Or, you may even smell gas as the underground pipes crack under the strain.

If you find yourself caught in a mudslide, do not run behind nearby homes or vehicles for cover. Make your way toward a clearing and move as far away from the sliding earth as you can. If you cannot escape it, lower your body and curl yourself into a ball protecting your head. After the mudslide settles down, move far away from the area, as there may be more that follows. Keep an eye out for fallen live power lines, ruptured sewer and gas lines, sharp debris, injured, buried and trapped people.

Now that you have had the chance to study the "Unlucky 7," you may want to develop counter-strategies for all those which affect your area of the country. They may devastate your home, leave you shaken, tired and weary, but if you are prepared, chances are you and your family will still be standing tall. In the final analysis, this is all that counts.

CHAPTER 19

"The Big One"
Earthquake
Volcano Eruption
Tsunami
Meteor
Preparedness

"THE BIG ONE IS COMING" TO THE UNITED STATES, SAY THE GEOLOGISTS. WHERE? WHEN? IT'S still an open question. The Indonesian megaquake of December 2004, that in turn created the tsunami that killed an estimated 300,000 people, once again shows us why we must prepare to help us survive the devastating effects of major natural catastrophes.

From most to least frequent, the following events are ones that we must recognize as a possible "big one" in our lives:

1. Earthquakes
2. Volcanic Eruptions
3. Tsunamis
4. Meteor Collision

You might believe that adding a "Meteor Collision" to this list is a bit far-fetched, but large collisions have happened many times in the past and will happen again. The meteor that exploded near Russia's Tunguska River in 1908 felled an estimated 60 million trees and a resulting column of fire rose thousands of feet into the air. If such a meteor struck a major city, the disaster would kill, wound and displace millions.

Among the list of "Big Ones," we will most likely confront large earthquakes and volcanic eruptions. Most of these occur within the "Ring of Fire," an area circling the Pacific Basin. Los Angeles and San Francisco sit precariously along its edges. Over the past decade, the frequency and magnitude of these quakes are increasing, indicating that we may be at the beginning of a frenzied quake cycle.

The year 2006 marks the centennial of the great San Francisco earthquake that demolished many of the city's buildings and sparked a huge fire, killing more than 2,500 people. The New York City area experienced a large earthquake estimated at 6.0 on the Richter scale in 1884. There have also been major earthquakes in Boston and Charleston, South Carolina.

The New Madrid fault zone of Missouri, Tennessee and Arkansas has seen three of the largest North American earthquakes in recorded history. Between 1811 and 1812, three earthquakes, judged by their aftermath to be at least 8.0 on the Richter scale, were so severe that they were felt across the entire country outside of the Pacific states. Entire meadows and homes were swallowed up, forests were destroyed, new lakes formed, and the course of the Mississippi river was altered. Scientists feel that another large earthquake above 6.0 on the Richter scale is certain to hit the New Madrid fault zone with a 90% chance of occurring by the year 2040.

Scientists have calculated a high probability of a large earthquake hitting Southern California in the next 30 years. If this quake is similar in size to the 1906 event in San Francisco, it could spawn a catastrophe that would dwarf the damage produced by Hurricane Katrina.

If you live around the Ring of Fire or the New Madrid zone, the most rational and prudent thing to do is formulate an earthquake survival plan as soon as possible. The Katrina tragedy has revealed that our government does not have the capability to respond to any major disaster. If any help comes, it may take weeks to arrive.

Earthquake Preparedness Essentials

Never leave home without your E-Kit. If you are ever caught in an earthquake, there is no way to predict where you will be, and whenever or wherever it hits, you must be ready to respond to it. The gear in your E-Kit will provide you with tools to do so properly. If you live in an earthquake-prone area, be sure to carry work gloves to protect your hands from being cut from glass and other debris, goggles, and a small first aid kit. Always wear comfortable shoes or at least have them nearby—if you are at work when the quake hits, you will be walking home, provided it is still there. Energy bars or trail mix are also great to carry for energy, a bottle of water and, if you really want to go hardcore, purchase a construction helmet and stash it under your desk or someplace near your work area where you can find it if and when the Big One hits.

The next step to take would be to prepare your home. Begin by making sure that everything in your home is anchored firmly to prevent it from falling and breaking.

- Bolt large cabinets, bookshelves, refrigerators, or any other large free-standing objects to the wall with metal angle brackets to wall studs. If you own a flat-screen television, you may want to run some stainless steel wire across the edges and screw it into the wall to anchor it more firmly. Fasten your water heater with plumbers tape (strap metal available at most good hardware stores) at the top, middle and bottom. This can prevent the heater from breaking free and possibly severing its gas line if you use natural gas.

- Fasten heavy-duty Velcro to every item in your home that can slide off of a shelf and break.
- Ceiling fans, chandeliers and other lighting fixtures can fall during earthquakes and cause serious injury. If you have them in your home, make sure they are mounted properly with earthquake safety wiring to prevent breakage and short circuits.
- If you have large mirrors or heavy artwork hanging in your home, do not mount them with nails. Use tongue-in-groove or screw-eyes hangers.
- Place tall furniture in areas of your home where it can't hit people if it falls.
- Do not place seating near items that can fall and injure.
- Place all large, heavy, fragile possessions on low shelves and install barrier wires to prevent objects from falling from shelves.
- Store hazardous items in cabinets that have good latches, like "swing hook" style latches.
- Move flammable material or flammable objects away from electrical wires.
- Repair all faulty wiring.
- Move emergency preparedness gear to an area where you could quickly grab it and run. This includes your fire extinguisher.
- Build a safe area free of furniture or any hazardous objects in your living room and bedrooms where you could stand or sit during an earthquake and not be hit by falling objects.
- If you have an infant, make sure that there are no objects that can fall into the crib and entrap, cut or injure the child. Move the crib away from electrical outlets or glass windows. Make sure there are no objects that can fall and block your path to the room. Do not place the crib under any hanging light or ceiling fan.
- Do not place any objects that could fall and block doors, windows or any other egress points.
- If you live in an old home with a basement, make certain that your floorboards are strong and your foundation is sturdy.
- If you use oxygen, the tanks must be firmly fastened to the wall. Keep canes or walkers nearby at all times. If possible, keep extras in the bathroom, kitchen and other areas of your home that you frequent.
- Make sure that every member of your home knows how and when to shut off your gas, electrical power and water.

- Put a battery-powered emergency light or lantern in every room in your home. Make sure that it is non-incendive.
- Use Venetian blinds or shades on all windows and keep them partially closed at all times as a barrier against breaking glass.
- If you have a gas dryer in your basement, make sure that it is bolted down securely and the flex gas cable is in good condition.
- If you have propane tanks attached to your home, make sure they are bolted down and all connections are secure.
- If you have a pet dog or cat, keep a travel cage handy along with extra food.

Earthquake Response

If You are Caught Indoors During an Earthquake:

- Find a sturdy table, desk, or bench and get under it to protect yourself from falling debris. If you are not near a table, desk or bench, grab a few chairs and slide underneath. If you are in bed, curl up in a fetal position and grab a pillow to protect your head. If you have time, and you can fit, crawl underneath. If you cannot do any of the above, stand against an inside wall without any hanging objects above, and hold your ground covering your head with your arms, or with a coffee table-sized book. Do not stand near windows, lights, artwork or heavy freestanding objects like refrigerators. If all the above options aren't possible, drop, cover your head and hang on.
- Wait a while before venturing outdoors. Aftershocks may dislodge falling debris.
- Don't depend upon a doorway as protection. Most of today's buildings are too flimsy and offer little protection.
- Never smoke during earthquakes. Ruptured gas mains and other flammable gases pose a serious threat, and smoking can put you and others at severe risk. Find the strength to curb your habit until the emergency is over.
- If you have children in your home, you must make a decision to run to them or wait out the first wave of the earthquake. If you run to them, you run the risk of injuring yourself. If you hurt yourself, you will not be in a condition to provide your children with the protection they will need to survive following the quake. Assess the situation carefully before making a move. If things look too dangerous, it is probably not a good

idea to try and reach them, although as a father of a young child, I know that I would without hesitation run through the devil's furnace to save my son. Whatever you decide to do choose wisely!

If You Are Caught Outdoors:

- Stand away from structures, utility poles, trees, lighting fixtures and manholes. If there is no clear area available you must make a judgment call and find a sturdy building to provide you with temporary shelter.
- If you are driving, slow down and be mindful of traffic. If you are driving over a bridge or overpass, get off at the next exit as quickly as possible. If you are in an underpass or tunnel, proceed rapidly (with caution) to the nearest exit.

IA TIP

If you see a wire wastebasket or large sturdy bucket nearby, turn it over and dump its contents on the street, and use it to protect your head from falling debris.

High-Rise Earthquake Preparedness and Escape

Earthquakes present a number of hazards for high-rise building tenants and workers: falling debris, fire, blackouts, elevator failure, communications break-downs, and gas and water leaks—especially if the high-rise is an older building with masonry fixtures.

- If you live in an earthquake-prone area, each family member or office worker should have safety helmets, goggles, and heavy-duty work gloves. They should be stashed next to your Grab-and-Go Bags, in desks or near entrances to apartments and offices.
- Each family member should have a particulate mask rated for protection against dust and mists (3M's are best), and goggles.
- Scoop stretchers should be placed near the first aid kit. Falling debris can produce injuries that require immobilization and rapid transportation. A lightweight scoop stretcher allows you to move injured co-workers safely and quickly.

High-rise workers and residents should drill regularly on earthquake safety and evacuation. The most important measures are:

- Move the injured and physically challenged first.
- Move away from large objects (*e.g.*, file cabinets and office machines) that could fall or crush.
- Move away from windows and elevator doors.
- Shelter yourself from falling debris under a strong table or desk.
- Use the stairway to evacuate your office.
- Once outside, quickly move away from the building. Seek cover from falling glass and other debris, and be wary of vehicular traffic, as falling debris may force drivers to drive erratically and endanger pedestrians.

Survival and escape from high-rise buildings during large fires and earthquakes requires a commitment to life on the part of those who live or work in them to learn how to use protective equipment and rehearse effective methods of escape.

When the Earthquake is Over:

- Check yourself and other family members for injuries, grab your emergency gear and leave your home with family if your structure is questionable.
- Prepare for aftershocks.
- If there is no power, do not use your flashlight unless it is of the non-incendive type. Do not use candles, flares or any type of flame-producing devices unless you are outdoors.
- Be conscious of fallen power lines and live wires.
- If damage to your home is severe, do not enter.
- Make sure to shut off your main gas valve.
- If you spot electrical damages, shut off your power at the circuit breaker or main fuse box.
- Don't use your flush toilets until you can confirm that your sewer lines are intact.
- If your home is relatively intact, enter and check for damages.
- Make sure that your phone is on the hook.
- Find shelter by nightfall and stay away from the streets, where you may encounter frightened animals, desperate people scrounging for food and water, and even armed looters.

Tsunamis

If you live near a coastline, you must watch for tsunamis after large earthquakes. One sure sign of a developing tsunami is a rapidly receding waterline around a beach that may extend more than a quarter mile. The waters can also rapidly rise. If you see this occurring, move quickly to a secure spot on high ground. Don't wait around to watch the phenomenon. Once you see the wave approaching, you won't have time to get away.

If a tsunami wave hits near where you live, grab hold of something that is rooted down like a strong tree or even a light pole. Lash yourself to this object with a belt or something similarly strong. Curl yourself around the object to avoid being knocked off by passing debris.

Volcanoes

Volcanic eruptions are not as common as earthquakes but they can produce tremendous amounts of damage, as they did during the Krakatoa of 1883, or during the unexpected 1943 eruption of the Paricutín volcano in a Mexican cornfield. The greatest danger from volcanic eruptions besides the obvious fiery lava can be the superheated volcanic ash. This is pulverized rock that is acrid, highly abrasive and acidic. It can spread out over wide areas from the eruption and can cause severe respiratory problems in children, the elderly and the ill. If you ever find yourself in the position of escaping a volcanic eruption, follow these basic rules:

- Move away from the site as quickly as possible.
- If the volcano is spitting out large amounts of ash, use your partial face respirator to help you to breathe. If you don't have a respirator, cover your mouth and nose with a piece of cloth. If you can find shelter, move inside and pay attention that the weight of the collecting ash doesn't cave in the roof.
- Look out for flying chunks of lava and rocks.
- Mudflows are a dangerous side effect from volcanic eruptions. If you see one approaching, move rapidly to higher ground if you cannot find a vehicle or even a bicycle to get away. Mudflows move at about 20 mph. It takes an Olympic-caliber sprinter to outrun it.
- If you live in a home that is a safe distance away from the eruption but the ash in your area is accumulating rapidly, you will need to keep all of your doors closed, shut down your air conditioner and close off

all ventilation grates. Stuff wet towels under your doors to prevent the ash from getting inside your home. The only device that I know of that wouldn't clog up and could help you keep the ash out of your air would be an air ionizer, but this is provided that you still have electrical power to run it.

■ Clear all ash buildup before it clogs up your storm drains.

■ Never drive during a volcanic eruption unless you are moving away to escape it. Try to avoid moving through areas with thick clouds of dust and ash. The abrasive qualities can ruin your car's engine.

■ Don't use appliances or electronic equipment near drifting ash clouds. The particulate can sometimes produce short circuits. You must also cover all of the vents on your computer, TV, stereo and other similar electronic devices. Do not use them until they are cleaned off.

If you are lucky, the closest that you will ever come to encountering the types of events mentioned in this chapter will be on a movie or television screen. If not, now you have a general understanding of what must be done to survive them.

CHAPTER 20

Infectious Disease

MODERN MEDICINE AND ITS TECHNICAL MARVELS MAY HAVE LULLED US INTO A FALSE SENSE of security about its ability to control deadly microorganisms that have plagued mankind for eons. Emerging diseases such as avian ("bird") flu, severe acute respiratory syndrome (SARS), hantavirus pulmonary syndrome and AIDS will produce misery and death for millions of people around the world while medical researchers struggle to find cures.

Preparedness calls for us to examine infectious diseases and how they are spread today. Crowded cities provide microorganisms with transmission mechanisms such as subways, buses, airports, rubbish, restaurants, food, shopping malls and transportation terminals. The ability of insects and pests to nest and proliferate in urban centers is another causal factor.

Consider the West Nile virus (WNV) in New York City. The virus was first identified in the city in 1999. Forty-five people were infected with it, and four died. To control the spread of WNV, local authorities began a controversial spray campaign using a toxic pesticide called Fyfanon ULV (Malathion) to kill the disease-carrying mosquitoes. Crop-dusting helicopters patrolled the city, spraying the pesticide on rooftops, streets, and people who didn't or couldn't move out of the way. WNV has shown up in more than ten eastern states since 1999 and shows no signs of slowing down. As travel, trade, and migration increase between tropical areas and our cities, WNV could soon be joined by more dangerous diseases such as malaria, eastern equine encephalitis, hantavirus, and Chagas disease (also known as urban yellow fever).

Common house pets are sources of contagion. Anywhere the animal sleeps or moves it leaves minute quantities of waste. If you walk your pet outside it will track small quantities of other animals' waste back inside. Animals also host disease-carriers such as ticks, fleas, and lice. Infants and the elderly are at especially high risk from infectious disease transmission by household pets. Puppies and kittens sometimes carry intestinal roundworms that are easily transmitted to infants. Even worse is potentially fatal cat-scratch infection. Zoonotic diseases—those transmitted from animals to humans—pose a threat to public health, especially where large numbers of animals and livestock live close to humans.

Zoonotic Diseases and Parasites	Animal Hosts
Plague	Rodents, cats (infected by rodents)
Roundworms (toxacariasis)	Cats, dogs
RVF (Rift Valley fever)	Dogs, cats
Psittacosis	Parrots, pigeons, parakeets, cockatiels
Toxoplasmosis	Cats
Cat scratch fever	Cats
Lice (e.g., scabies)	Humans, dogs, cats, cattle, horses,
Rabies	Dogs, cats, raccoons, bats, cattle, horses, beavers
Hookworm	Dogs
Hantavirus	Rodents
Q-Fever	Cats
Campylobacteriosis	Cats, dogs
Lyme disease	Wild rodents, deer
Ringworm (dermatophytosis)	Dogs, horses, cats
Leptospirosis	Dogs
Systemic fungal disease	Dogs, cats, pigeons
Small roundworms (strongyloidiasis)	Dogs, cats
Giardia	Dogs
Mange (mites)	Dogs, cats
Cryptosporidium	Cattle
Tapeworm (echinococcosis)	Dogs, horses

These combined dangers illustrate the need for a personal infectious disease protection program. Controlling the spread of infectious disease is a major concern for the health departments of the world's largest cities and should also be the individual's concern.

How to Protect Yourself from Infectious Diseases in Urban Areas

The first step in any urban infectious disease protection program is controlling your levels of exposure. In a city, the areas of highest risk are:

■ Large crowds in tight spaces with poor ventilation—*e.g.*, subways and subway stations, buses, house parties, offices.
■ Hospital emergency rooms.
■ Crowded restaurants (transmission via food).
■ Supermarkets, malls, cinemas, large stores (many large record stores have listening stations with headphones that are never cleaned, putting listeners at risk for head lice).
■ Churches. The worst large-scale emergencies tend to send people flocking to churches, many of which are poorly ventilated.
■ Garbage collection areas—risk increases as frequency of collection decreases.
■ Workplace: health-care workers have an elevated risk of exposure. Train conductors, police officers, paramedics, trash collectors, taxi drivers and waiters are also at higher risk.

To Reduce Risk of Disease

■ Wash your hands. Carry a small pack of sanitary wipes for when you are not near a washroom. Maintaining clean hands is a simple and highly effective measure against communicable diseases.
■ If you regularly handle items touched by many people (*e.g.*, coin and paper money, utensils, subway grips), wear latex or nitrile gloves.
■ Use protection during sexual contact.
■ Thoroughly wash all food, and use clean cutting boards and utensils—disinfected after contact with fish, poultry, or meat and before contact with any other food. A solution of bleach in water (about 1 tbsp/quart) works well.

- Do not share cigarettes, straws, etc.
- When using public toilets, try not to touch the doorknobs or toilet flusher handle. Use a paper towel, your shirt, or some other barrier.
- Make sure that any restaurant food you eat is prepared by workers wearing protective gloves.
- If you are a trash collector or subway conductor make particulate respirators and puncture-resistant Kevlar gloves part of your standard operating gear.

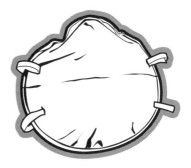

3M N95 Mask

Use the particulate respirators suited to your occupation. Garbage collectors, train conductors (due to contact with steel dust) and those who handle medical waste need a 3M variety R-95 to R or P-100 respirator.
- When riding crowded subways and buses during flu season, wear a 3M N95-100 respirator.
- Avoid vendors at unfamiliar restaurants and street carts who are not wearing plastic gloves. When ordering pizza, make sure that it is piping hot. Stay away from questionable seafood and open buffets.
- If you are hospitalized and notice that a doctor or nurse fails to wash hands and wear gloves while preparing to change an IV or conduct some other contact medical procedure, politely request that he or she do so, and if this is refused, call for another nurse or doctor. Don't worry about hurting anyone's feelings. Every hospital has a patient's bill of rights, and you have the right to request another nurse or physician if you feel jeopardized by carelessness.
- Wash or wipe off the tops of cans before opening them.
- Beware of public beaches and pools. Polluted water can transmit a variety of illnesses that endanger children, the elderly, and people with compromised immune systems. Swimmers in polluted water risk contracting hepatitis, *E. coli,* respiratory illnesses, swimmer's ear, gastroenteritis, and many other dangerous diseases. The Natural Resources Defense Council estimates that over 40% of all American beaches are too polluted for safe swimming. Public beaches are also polluted with other hazards such as medical waste, human and other feces, and trash. When walking on public beaches, wear sneakers or thick sandals.
- If you eat in fast-food restaurants, don't let your food touch the trays, which are rarely cleaned thoroughly.

- At health clubs, wipe gym machines clean before using them. Avoid public hot tubs, which can pass diseases such as staphylococcus, Legionnaire's disease, Pontiac fever, skin diseases, and eye and ear infections.
- Police officers and journalists are advised to carry extra protection with their E-Kits, including: a protective suit (chemical and biological—or level C), a particulate respirator, goggles, a safety helmet, and puncture- and chemical-resistant gloves. 3M's SCBAG (Self-Contained Breathing Apparatus) kit contains two sets of Tyvek F coveralls with attached hood and boots, two pairs of haz-mat booties, and two pairs of protective gloves. This kit can protect you from a variety of chemical and biological hazards you may encounter during an emergency response.
- If you are a cyclist, carry the bicycle when you enter and leave your house or apartment instead of rolling the tires on the floor.
- Remove your shoes when entering your home.
- Never share make-up.

Pet Owners

- Never let your pet roam freely outside. Pets that roam have a greater chance of being exposed to diseased animals.
- Do not allow small children to play with pets unsupervised. Children tend to allow pets near their faces, and to not wash their hands after handling animals. Dangerous diseases such as salmonella (from turtles) can be passed on by this behavior.
- Wash the area where your pet sleeps, eats and leaves its waste.
- Make sure that your pet is vaccinated against rabies and other diseases. Kittens and puppies should be treated for intestinal worms.
- Do not let your pet play near the trash.
- Stay away from unfamiliar animals.
- Don't buy exotic pets that belong in their natural habitats and not in your home. When ill, exotic pets tend to transmit exotic diseases.
- After walking a dog in the rain, wash his paws with mild soap and dry them before letting him roam your home.
- Wash your hands as soon as possible after contact with any animal.
- Learn how to spot the symptoms of rabies. If your pet becomes skittish or aggressive and begins to drool, take it to a veterinarian or call an animal control officer. If a pet bites you, seek immediate medical attention.

Insect Control

Urban insect control requires integrated pest management systems and clean-up campaigns that clear out areas where mosquitoes and other pests live and breed: junkyards, vacant lots, and tire dumps, among others.

- Empty mini-pools in your backyards when they aren't being used.
- Clear your rooftop's drains.
- Dispose of old tires that collect rainwater: mosquitoes use them as hatcheries.
- Seal up your garbage before leaving it on the street.

Pandemic Preparedness Protocols

Experts say we are probably on the brink of a global pandemic similar to the 1918 Spanish Flu epidemic that killed 675,000 Americans and 50–100 million others around the world. The projected U.S. death toll of a moderate pandemic would be more than one-half million. More than two million people would need to be hospitalized and almost 67 million Americans will be sickened according to the Washington, D.C.-based Trust for America's Health. A severe outbreak could produce from 700,000 to three million fatalities.

With an outbreak of any virus (swine flu, avian flu, etc.), vaccines would eventually be produced in limited quantities. It would be steady, but not fast enough to inoculate the entire U.S. population in time to prevent large numbers of illnesses and deaths. Mexico, Latin America, and the Carribbean (with the exception of Puerto Rico and the U.S. Virgin Islands) do not have the resources to produce vaccines, and would be socially and economically devastated by a pandemic. In early 2009, the swine flu shut down Mexico City, and had an enormous impact on tourism and other aspects of the Mexican economy.

A full-blown pandemic would have catastrophic long-term consequences for the entire region. Our nation will likely become a three-million-square-mile hot zone with large cities quarantined by the military operating under strict COG (Continuity of Government) laws designed to maintain order.

There are things you can do prior to a pandemic to avoid becoming its victim.

The only medicine that has been deemed even somewhat effective in treating avian flu is Tamiflu (oseltamivir). It has been shown to be useful in some cases when taken before serious illness develops but the H5N1 strain is showing signs that it may be developing a resistance. A number of patients in Asia who were given Tamiflu died during treatment. This recent development is forcing many governments around the world to rethink their avian flu strategies. Tamiflu will not be enough to combat this highly virulent virus, which will take a combination of methods to help keep it under control. To combat avian flu:

- Make your body as inhospitable to flu viruses as possible. Modify your diet to include as many flu-fighting foods and beverages as possible. The fermented Korean cabbage dish called *kimchi* has shown some promise after a study by scientists in Seoul discovered that 11 of 13 chickens infected with avian flu recovered after they were fed an extract of *kimchi*. Dark grape juice, filled with tannins, may help to keep the virus under control. Tannins have been known to kill flu viruses in laboratories. Elderberry is also showing promise.

IA TIP

Never use elderberry unless it is the commercially produced extract. The flowers, unripe berries, bark, roots, leaves contain cyanide. Look for elderberry capsules, juice, syrup, in your local health food store.

- Be alert—pay attention to all related news reports. If you hear about any suspicious illnesses in your building, neighborhood or place of employment, inquire about the illness, and who was infected so you can avoid contact with them.
- During an outbreak, if you travel by train or bus to work or school, use a partial face respirator of the N-100 class—nothing less. Do not be embarrassed about looking strange. You will look even stranger if you contract the flu.
- Keep a large supply of non-perishable food items and water stocked away in your home during winter months. For a pandemic, you would need at least a month. This will cut back on the need for traveling to grocery stores. In addition, this will also allow you to stay inside your home just in case your area becomes quarantined.
- If you use public laundromats to wash your clothes, use a disinfectant (Lysol or anything of industrial strength) to clean out the washing machine. Detergent does not kill flu viruses.

- If you frequently use taxis, be sure to ride with the window down. If you want to be safe, use that partial face respirator. When you leave the cab, use your antibacterial hand cleanser.
- Do not sit on your bed sheets in your street clothes.
- Take Vitamin C every day; some recommend megadoses against avian flu. There is no comprehensive study to confirm this but some invoke the 1949 case of Dr. Frederick Klenner, a clinical researcher from Reidsville, North Carolina, who infused 60 polio patients with massive intravenous doses of Vitamin C–20,000 mg daily for three days. After the treatment and a period of rest, all 60 were cured. If you are ever infected with avian flu, and your treatments are unsuccessful, it may be your physician's best last-resort method to try the Vitamin C cure.
- Wash hands frequently during an outbreak. This is one of the best methods to prevent infection.
- Purchase a humidifier for your home and use it during flu season to keep your home from becoming too dry.
- Avoid touching your eyes, nose and mouth.
- Avoid restaurants, malls, department stores, coffee shops or any public gathering area until the outbreak is under control. When traveling in high-traffic areas, keep your respirator mask on and carry plenty of hand sanitizer. If you must use public bathrooms, clean your hands with sanitizer after touching any surface.

A global pandemic will force us to consider drastic changes in our lifestyle. They will be difficult to deal with but are a more tolerable alternative than contracting a disease with a mortality rate that fluctuates between fifty and one hundred percent.

CHAPTER 21

Chemical and Bio-Warfare

THE INTENTIONAL OR ACCIDENTAL RELEASE OF CHEMICAL OR BIOLOGICAL AGENTS IN A MAJOR city can produce a large number of fatalities and serious injuries. Prepared people must understand what these agents are and what they can do.

Biological agents are difficult to detect. You cannot distinguish them with any of your five senses. The first sign of a biological agent will be symptoms of the victims exposed to the agent. The five types of bioweapons are:

- Microorganisms—viruses, fungi, protozoa, bacteria, rickettsiae.
- Vectors—insects, animals, reptiles, birds.
- Plant and animal pests.
- Anti-crop agents and herbicides.
- Toxins.

Biological weapons may be used because they have the following critical advantages over other types of weaponry:

- Their relative cheapness to manufacture, especially compared to nuclear weapons.
- Manufacturing plants and dissemination systems can be easily disguised or hidden.
- Bio-agents can be disseminated over large areas. Cities and their concentrated populations are particularly vulnerable.
- Bio-agents are difficult to defend against.

The most efficient method of delivery for biological material is by aerosol mist with commonly available fumigation devices and chemicals. The biological agent is mixed with a base that allows it to be sprayed in a fine mist with particles around two microns in size. Larger particles drop to the ground quickly because of their weight. Tiny droplets quickly reach the bloodstream.

Bio-Weapon Dissemination Methods

Attacks would take place in the late evening—for the cover of darkness—or during the morning rush hours, to maximize direct exposure. Dissemination can occur in various ways:

Vehicle: Devices can be disguised as exhaust pipes on automobiles, trains, boats, trucks, or incinerator chimneys.

Air: Crop-dusting planes and helicopters can contaminate large areas with infectious material. An aerial attack would most likely take place in the early morning in late summer or early fall. This could be conducted by a terrorist flying a crop-duster a few hundred feet above ground in a zig-zag path. Under the right conditions, this method could deliver an infectious dose to 30,000 people. If you spot an aircraft flying slowly and spraying, quickly move away from the area. (It may just be an insecticide, but insecticides aren't safe, either.)

Water: Large cities depend on reservoirs for their water supply. Due to poor security around important areas in water delivery systems—pumping stations, control valves, and filtration/purification stations—city water supplies are vulnerable to biological and chemical weapons attacks. Toxins such as botulinum toxin type A would be the biological agents of choice for this type of attack. Ounce for ounce, this is the most poisonous organic substance on earth.

The technique most likely employed by terrorists to poison a water supply is called "backflow." This method uses modified water or bicycle pumps (even a industrial vacuum cleaner) to push dangerous chemicals, toxins or biological material into local water distribution systems. This method could contaminate water for many thousands of people in any given area of a city or town.

If a large city's drinking water supply were contaminated, limited supplies of potable water would be distributed by the National Guard, Red Cross, FEMA, and other disaster relief agencies. Because of the large demand and inadequate delivery methods for such a crisis, many areas would be overlooked and neglected. Explosive social situations would result.

By hand: a finely-powdered form of anthrax could be delivered by a single individual armed with small quantities in glass vials or bottles. They could be dumped into air conditioning and ventilation systems of large buildings, or simply thrown onto subway tracks. The passing trains would act as pistons pushing the material through tunnels for miles.

Highly contagious and robust viruses and other dangerous microorganisms can also be delivered on commonly used objects and materials. Food, carpets in public areas or any commonly contacted surface that is shielded from direct sunlight (sunlight kills most dangerous bacteria) would do. A terrorist could contaminate almost anything with certain types of bacteria and viruses, including:

■ Paper currency and coins.
■ Candy, canned and frozen food (during production).
■ Public bathrooms, benches, tables, doorknobs, subway door handles, turnstiles, gas station pumps, mail.
■ Bus and subway poles.
■ Elevator buttons.
■ Escalator railings.
■ Newspapers.
■ Mock junk mail.
■ Cigarette packages/cigarettes.
■ Envelopes or stamps (the glue can be laced with the agent).
■ Paper towels in public restrooms.

These all may seem unlikely ways to infect a city with bio-warfare, but Al Qaeda war manuals show how to use bio-weapons to contaminate the things listed above.

Terrorists may attempt to spread anthrax, plague, cholera, or less familiar viruses. Possible pathogens range from those that tend to kill infected persons quickly (such as Ebola fever) to those that can inflict years of misery (such as brucellosis). Since there are so many possibilities for bio-terrorism—or accidents leading to disastrous releases of the same agents—your preparedness plan should take a preventive approach aimed at common features of the multitude of agents. During the last stages of the Cold War, the Russian Biopreparat designed a biological weapons strike against New York City that included more than 27 types of agents.

The destructive power of a biological agent depends on a number of conditions. People with compromised immune systems are particularly vulnerable. Poor communities in large cities are densely populated and have large amounts of uncollected rubbish and vacant dilapidated buildings—breeding grounds for vermin and insects that can serve as vectors for disease. In addition, many residents do not have medical insurance. Millions more are undocumented and live in fear of the INS. If they happen to get exposed to and contract an infectious "weaponized" biological agent such as smallpox, it is highly unlikely that they will seek medical attention when they begin to manifest symptoms. This is a critical period when the disease can be spread from aerosolized saliva droplets expelled from the mouth when coughing, sneezing or even talking.

To make matters worse, many undocumented immigrants work in agriculture and restaurant industries where they are in contact with food and people. These conditions may well be exploited by the bioterrorist.

Bio-Warfare Preparedness

Of all available dissemination methods, inhalation of aerosolized agents is the most lethal. Agents that settle in the lungs cannot be exhaled, and continue to produce damage even after you have left the contaminated area. This is why it's so important to include 3M particulate respirators in your E-Kit and Grab-and-Go Bag. Uncovered eyes can also be injured by some bio-weapons and provide infection portals for others. Thus the suggestion for carrying eye goggles in your Grab-and-Go Bag.

Large buildings and heavy vehicular traffic produce wind currents at street level to move contaminated air. As the wind blows, toxicity is diminished, but it's still dangerous if inhaled or absorbed through broken skin. This is why lip balm belongs in your E-Kit: germs can enter the body through chapped lips. Weather also plays a role in transmission; high humidity, for example, speeds absorption through skin.

Integrating the following suggestions into your daily life can help you prepare for the possibility of bio-warfare and other sorts of attacks and accidents:

- Stay alert! Learn to notice apparent cold and flu outbreaks. Initial symptoms caused by bio-warfare agents can mimic common ailments. If you begin to see large numbers of others with cold or flu-like symptoms, see a doctor immediately. If you have been exposed to anthrax, your time for treatment is limited. Large doses of antibiotics can destroy the organism—but once you have begun to manifest symptoms, it may be too late for treatment.
- Avoid crowds. Large gathering areas (stadiums, terminals, subway stations) are the most likely targets of bio-terrorists. Subway users should try to arrange their schedules to use the trains before and after the rush hours.
- Install water filters/distillers. Potable water is your highest priority. Make sure that you have a high-quality unit in your home that can be used in the event of a bio-weapon attack. The only micro-organisms that cannot be filtered out are viruses, which are too small for most filters. All houses should have a robust emergency water supply with no less than a seven-day minimum.
- Avoid eating from open buffets. They're easy targets.

- Avoid fast-food or large-volume restaurants.
- Thoroughly wash all of your food and utensils. Remove vegetable skins before eating.
- Remove shoes before entering your home. Have a mat to wipe your shoes and a mat where they can be placed. Removing shoes reduces the chance of tracking potentially dangerous biological material into your living space.
- Carpets are magnets for dirt, dust, airborne contaminants. Remove them if you can.
- Houseplants can oxygenate and filter the air in your home.
- Purchase air filters and ionizers to help keep your air clean during a bio-weapon attack (provided you still have electrical power or off-grid power sources).
- Seal up your home. Inspect all of your windows' and doors' rubber seals; check your ventilation systems for mold, dust, and other blockages; seal off any drafty areas.

If You Are Caught at Home During a Bio-Weapons Incident

Improvised air filters can cover vents, air conditioner ports, dryer vents, fireplaces, and other points of entry. You will need the following materials:

- Construction-grade duct tape or gaffers tape.
- Insect wire mesh screens in three-foot-square sheets to be later cut to the sizes of all air vents.
- HEPA replacement filters. The following HEPA filters should fit over a typical apartment air vent grate: Hamilton Beach TrueAir replacement filters for the 04162, 04163, and 04912 air cleaning units; Bionaire A1230H replacement filter for the BAP1175 and BAP1300 air cleaners; the Vornado MD-1004 replacement filter for the AQ25 and AQS35 air cleaners, or any other HEPA filter that fits.

To Construct An Improvised Vent Assembly:

Cut insect screen to size, place it over the vent, and tape down the edges with duct tape. The HEPA filter goes on top of the insect screen, taped down, with all edges thoroughly inspected for gaps. The covered vents are temporary emergency measures designed to filter your air for up to ten days.

- Clean hands are your first line of defense against contamination. A good hand-washing with warm water and soap can effectively eliminate up to 98% of harmful bacteria. Keep your fingernails short and clean.
- Avoid unnecessary travel. If you must travel, wear a gas mask (or full face respirator rated for organic mists) and protective clothing.
- Keep antibiotics on hand. I suggest that you make an appointment with your doctor now and have a frank conversation about this important topic and request a prescription for Cipro, amoxicillin, or broad-spectrum antibiotics. You need to learn what the recommended daily doses should be for you, your children or elderly family members.

If your doctor won't help you, find another who will. This is a grave matter that must be taken seriously. Our system is not prepared to handle a massive biological attack. It doesn't have the resources or manpower and even worse, the response plans are flawed. You must take matters into your own hands now.

When I interviewed Dr. Ken Alibek, author of *Biohazard* and former director of the huge Russian bio-warfare research program called Biopreparat, I asked him about the distribution of antibiotic medications and his reply was, "The Department of Health and Human Services says to us, 'we've got antibiotics stockpiled and if something happens, we would be able to provide antibiotics within the next 24 to 48 hours.' But, you know, I don't believe that I would be able to get those antibiotics within 24 hours—and I want my children alive."

This is from a man who helped to design some of the most lethal bio-weapons imaginable and is now working at George Mason University to help protect our nation from future bio-warfare attacks. Dr. Alibek understands better than anyone the consequences of a large-scale bio-warfare strike. Citizens need to be bold enough to grab the bull by the horns and stock protective antibiotic agents against a biowarfare breakout.

Chemical Weapons

Chemical weapons are of three types: harassing, incapacitating, and lethal. Harassing agents, such as tear gas, produce teary eyes, violent coughing, vomiting in exposed persons. Most people exposed to harassing agents will recover quickly after they leave the area of release.

People exposed to incapacitating agents will suffer more severe effects, and many will need rapid medical attention. Finally, nerve weapons such as VX, tabun, and sarin kill on contact or from inhalation.

The toxicity of any chemical agent varies with:

1. The individual health of the exposed person.
2. The purity of the substance.
3. The concentration in the air.

A harassing or incapacitating agent can be lethal if the exposed person suffers from poor health or if the concentrations in the area of release are high. A lethal agent may be reduced to a harassing agent if the concentrations in the air and purity levels are low, and the resistance of the affected person is high.

Inhalation is the most dangerous form of exposure to a chemical agent, as the lungs quickly absorb the agent and spread it through the entire body. Chemical weapons can also be absorbed cutaneously, and contact with chemical agents such as mustard gas will damage the skin as it is absorbed into the body. It's important to keep your body covered in an area where chemical weapons have been released.

Durability of the threat depends on the agent used. Nerve weapons such as VX and lewisite are called "persistent agents," remaining effective in a deployment area for weeks. Such weapons can contaminate subway stations, vehicles, and even food. Other agents will break up within a few hours or days after being released.

Nerve agents work directly on the central nervous system by blocking the production of an enzyme (cholinesterase) in the brain that regulates and controls breathing.

The most dangerous chemical weapons a terrorist group might use are:

- Choking gas: CG, phosgene
- Blood gas: AC, hydrogen cyanide
- Blister gas: H, mustard gas
- Lewisite
- Tabun (GA)
- Sarin (GB)
- Soman (GD)
- VX
- Cyclosarin (GF)
- VR
- Medimo
- Novichok
- Agent 33

Probable Targets:

- Transportation terminals.
- Subways and other mass transit.
- Sports events, concerts, special events, movie theaters.
- Shopping malls.
- Food supplies.

Protection Against Chemical Weapons

Preparation for chemical attacks is tricky. Your survival depends upon what the agent is and how much exposure you've had. A good way to protect yourself is to cover up as much of you body as possible in crowded areas. Chemical weapons are contact poisons. The more surface area of your skin that is exposed, the higher the degree of contamination. You should also pay close attention to others nearby. If you see large amounts of people rubbing their eyes, move away from the area quickly.

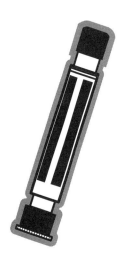

Atropine Auto-Injector

Always carry a smoke escape hood and a jacket with you in case an agent is released. A windbreaker made of Gore-Tex or PVC-coated nylon is best. But if you want the ultimate in chemical weapon protection, get an atropine auto-injector kit.

You would have to learn how to use the atropine injector properly, and unfortunately this takes training only available in EMT courses and in the military.

Biological and chemical weapons are among the most brutal weapons ever devised. Since their first recorded use in 1346 by the Mongol Tartars against the residents of Fedosia, they have been a plague upon our species. The right defensive skills will help protect you from their awful effects if you are ever unlucky enough to be among their targets.

CHAPTER 22

Nuclear/ Radiological Event Preparedness

Nuclear Terrorism

THE MOST DANGEROUS FORM OF TERRORISM INVOLVES THE USE OF NUCLEAR OR RADIOLOGICAL weapons. Nuclear bombs kill by blast, heat, radiation, and when the faint of heart see a mushroom cloud, by fear as well. Radiological weapons—or "dirty bombs"—are conventional explosives laced with radioactive material.

When detonated, radioactive material is pulverized into a fine powder that is distributed by wind currents. This can contaminate large regions of land, rendering them uninhabitable. It will also create long-term health problems for the unfortunate people who inhale or come into contact with the highly toxic dust.

Horrific as these weapons are, you can protect yourself from their effects. If you live through the initial shock wave, heat flash and dust cloud from a dirty bomb blast without being incapacitated, the following information will help you know how to minimize exposure to lethal fallout and how to survive until help arrives.

SADM (Special Atomic Demolition Munition) or Improvised Nuclear Device

If terrorists go nuclear, this is the weapon most likely to be used. Most SADMs would detonate to a tenth of the size of the Hiroshima bomb—still equivalent to 1,000 tons of dynamite in blast force. The rules to survive the effects stay the same no matter the size of the blast, though damage and fallout increase with blast power.

A one kiloton SADM ground burst in a crowded city would likely produce 20,000–100,000 fatalities from the blast, heat, radiation, structural failures, debris, and large gas fires ignited by the detonation. Five to ten city blocks would be destroyed. Basements and subway stations near the blast would be flooded by water main ruptures. Gas lines near the blast would also be broken, and burning cars and other material on the street would trigger gas explosions and, as a result, larger fires in surrounding structures.

The detonation's electromagnetic pulse would travel along power lines and antennas disabling communications devices, computers, automobiles and sensitive solid-state electronic equipment in the vicinity of the blast.

Fallout levels from SADMs are lower than from more powerful nuclear explosives, but are dangerous nevertheless. Weather conditions will determine the direction and coverage of the fallout cloud. Large areas of surrounding territory could be contaminated.

In the event of a nuclear blast, even SADM-sized, the nation's emergency response apparatus would be taxed to its limit. All medical establishments would operate from emergency triage guidelines, passing over the injured for the most critical cases. In some areas, important medications might not be available. Blood will also be scarce. Many severely injured patients will be left unattended because limited resources will leave no way to help them.

Food will be in short supply, and severe infrastructural damage and fallout will mean water shortages in some areas. Electrical power will be intermittent or unavailable for long periods. Communications will be disrupted. Disease will spread because of unburied rotting corpses and fallout-weakened immune systems. Crime may go unchecked.

Nuclear Missile Attack

The second nuclear event scenario is an ICBM (Intercontinental Ballistic Missile) attack—an improbable but possible event. The only countries equipped to blast an international target are the United States, France, United Kingdom, Russia, China and North Korea. Out of that group, only North Korea is considered a serious threat to conduct a nuclear strike against the United States. A catastrophic failure of the command control and communications systems that control our nuclear arsenals, a dreadful accident or deliberate launch provoked by conflict are the other ways a nuclear strike would be initiated.

Recent changes in U.S. policy regarding the use of nuclear weapons have made this frightening scenario more possible. The newly revised Doctrine for Joint Nuclear Operations allows the President to order a nuclear strike on a country that is said to harbor or support terrorists planning to use chemical or biological weapons against the United States. Russian President Vladimir Putin recently announced to the world that his military is in possession of an ICBM that can fly in a "zig zag" pattern. Defense Minister Sergei Ivanov declares, "There is not now and will not be any defense from such missiles."

It may seem obvious, but it bears stating that radiation is invisible, and the only way to tell you have been exposed to it is by testing yourself with a radiation dosimeter. I carry one with me at all times. The EPA has a unit called the Environmental Radiation Ambient Monitoring System, or ERAMS for short.

The EPA is charged with the task of reporting radiation levels to emergency management groups in your district. The problem here is that the intensity of ground-level radiation may vary significantly from area to area. The only way to know if you are in a safe zone is to measure the levels yourself. You will need a radiation detection device, and the best one available for civilians is called a Nukalert, a radiation detection alarm that chirps when exposed to anything radioactive. It is small and designed to be worn on a keychain.

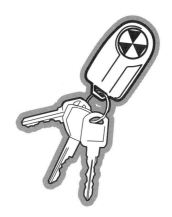

Nukalert

The Nukalert (www.NukAlert.com) costs $160 and gives you an instant warning about radiation levels in your area. It is calibrated to cheep more frequently when exposed to higher radiation levels. I consider this device a must-have item for anyone in the United States that lives in or near a large city or nuclear power plant.

More sophisticated radiation detection devices are called dosimeters or radiation dose rate meters. They range in price between $70 and $1,000 for high-end professional units. A dose rate meter is simple to read if you are familiar with the different radiation units of measurement (examined later in this chapter). Some devices have meters similar to voltimeters or analog automobile speedometers on the front or at the top of the units. Others have digital displays that display the radiation levels on LCD screens.

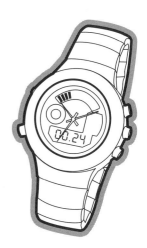

**GammaMaster
Dosimeter Watch**

Nuclear Event Survival Protocols

An accident or terrorist attack at a nuclear power plant can result in a full or partial meltdown. It doesn't matter which situation you encounter. Nuclear detonations and "dirty bombs" require a few extra special response protocols. The following list covers the most important rules:

- If you see a suspicious flash like lightning, duck and cover immediately. This advice may bring to mind the infamous civil defense film, *Duck and Cover.* The film may be antique, but it pays to heed its advice. The blast from even a small tactical nuclear device will turn glass shards into miniature flying buzzsaws and pebbles into buckshot. If you are relatively close to the point of detonation, ducking and covering is the only way to keep yourself from becoming a piece of human confetti. If you are standing near a window, immediately turn your back and drop to the floor covering your head.
- If you are nearby or downwind of a large conventional explosion, assume that it is laced with radioactive material. Prepare to take protective measures, which includes using partial face respirators to protect you from the inhalation of smoke. If you do not have one handy, cover your nose and mouth with a cloth or towel. swimmers' goggles are great eye protection. They are inexpensive and can be easily carried in your pocket. Keep your hair covered; if it becomes contaminated, you may be ordered to shave it off. Many commonly-used hair products will trap particulate matter in your hair. Once you get to a safe area, carefully dispose of your hat or whatever you used to cover your head in a plastic bag.

IA TIP

If you use swimmers' goggles, do not remove them until you are completely clear of the danger area. If you take them off in a contaminated zone, they will trap particulate matter inside.

- Find a water source and wet the towel or cloth to create a moisture barrier that can help trap particulate. Use this same source to collect a supply of drinking water that you can bottle up and take with you if you need to evacuate, or store away if you plan to stay where you are.
- With "dirty bombs", the concentration of radioactive material will be significantly less (outside of the immediate blast area) than a nuclear detonation and will allow for a safer evacuation.

Nuclear detonations produce very heavy concentrations of highly radioactive fallout that can produce lethal doses upwards of 500/rems in one hour.

■ If you are close to the most seriously damaged areas, you will probably not have enough time to escape the fallout cloud. Find a thick-walled steel-reinforced concrete structure and hunker down inside, getting behind as many walls as possible between you and areas where fallout would collect. In other words, stay clear of places like rooftops, terraces, courtyards. If you are in a home, gather your supplies, including as much water as you can find, extra food, a bucket and plastic bags for human waste disposal. Then close all of your doors, stuffing clothing underneath to prevent wind currents inside of your home from blowing around the fallout. Move to the room with the thickest walls to provide the best protective barriers against any collecting fallout. If you have a basement, move to the deepest point.

Use large cabinets, closet doors, boxes and what you can find to build a small covered and contained area large enough for you (and your family) to crawl inside. This will provide extra barriers against the radiation. Keep your food, water and toilet close enough to grab and pull into the makeshift structure. This makeshift accommodation will be an uncomfortable arrangement, but it can dramatically reduce the risks of contracting radiation sickness. Don't forget to keep your respirator mask on.

Listen for information on your radio for local news or the Emergency Alert System. If you don't have a radio available, just stay put. Radiation levels will drop enough in about seven days to safely escape from the area and seek help.

If you have the ability to move away from the contaminated area right after the blast, you must first check the wind direction by observing the orientation of the expanding smoke cloud, or if you are in an open area away from buildings, hold a tissue, handkerchief, or piece of newspaper over your head and observe the direction that the wind blows it. Take three measurements to make certain of the breeze's consistency. Once this is established, move in the opposite direction from the wind. This is the best way to ensure that you are moving away from the fallout if you do not have a radiation detection device (Nukalert) or accurate information from the local authorities.

Put on a raincoat or jacket, if you have it, as barrier between you and the radioactive dust. Even a large trash bag can help to protect you. Cut a hole in the bottom for your head and two on the side for your arms, and slip it on like a coat to keep dust and smoke out of your clothing and away from any open sores or cuts. If you cannot move out of the area quickly enough to escape the fallout cloud, seek shelter immediately and use the sheltering instructions to protect yourself from the radiation.

If you get any dust in your eyes, wash it out with water, or better yet, an eyewash solution. Carry the kind of eyewash that comes with a cup to put over your eye in your first aid kit. Wyeth Laboratories makes a good unit complete with eyewash cup called "soothing collyrium for fresh eyes eyewash." Carry it in your first aid kit.

Pets exposed to the smoke and dust will also need to be thoroughly washed or shaved. Any pet with hair or feathers must be decontaminated. You will probably need to take the animals to a veterinarian to have this done properly. Sadly, most of our pets will not survive a nuclear emergency.

Food exposed to the smoke and dust must be discarded. The general rule is: if it's not in a can, it's not safe.

If You Self-Decontaminate, Observe These Rules:

Once you reach a safe area, you need to decontaminate yourself. Doing this properly will require a change of clothes, shoes, trash bags, clean water source, hose, paper, pen, tape, bucket (if a shower is not available), detergent, and a pair of rubber gloves (dishwashing gloves will do).

Keep your nose, eyes and hair covered while you cautiously remove your clothing. Start with your shoes and work your way up. Keep your respirator mask on as you put the contaminated clothing inside a plastic bag. After you bag all the clothes, slowly seal it up. Alert waste disposal teams by writing a note about its radioactive contents, and then tape it to the bag.

Do not put on clean clothes until you are thoroughly cleaned off. Your change of clothing and shoes should remain sealed until ready to use.

Mix detergent with water and lather yourself from head to toe; wash yourself like you never have before, including underneath your fingernails. Do not scrub hard, just gently wipe the soap away. Completely rinse the soap from your body, especially your hair. Pay special attention to clean any open sores or cuts. Use hydrogen peroxide to clean out minor lacerations or bruises.

Clothing exposed to the smoke and dust must be discarded, along with drapes, curtains, bed sheets, tablecloths, and other items made from fabric. Dispose of clothing and other fabric items in plastic bags with a note regarding the contents' radioactivity.

Anything exposed to the dust and smoke cloud should be discarded.

Protection for Children

If you have school-age children and do not live or work within walking distance of their school, you will need to provide them with protective items they can use to cover their bodies and prevent the inhalation of radioactive particulate. They must either carry the following gear to school every day or have it set up at the school itself.

PVC Rainsuit. This is an inexpensive item that can be found practically everywhere. They come in their own plastic bags and can be packed away in their backpacks or briefcases. The best types to purchase are those that have elastic in the legs and arms to prevent moisture (or dust) from seeping in. In the event of a nuclear emergency, you must teach them to put it on, and keep it on until they are removed from the contaminated area.

Partial Face Respirators. Kimberly-Clark makes a children's mask with Mickey Mouse and other Disney characters on the front. Older children will need a small sized N-95 or N-100 mask. This mask is available from most medical supply stores. Your children must be instructed on how to put it on properly and to keep it on until they are taken into a safe area. I taught my son how to put on his partial face respirator when he was three years old, right after we both watched the second plane crash into the World Trade Center. He took to it right away and learned how to put it on and keep it on.

They also need a water bladder. The Camelbak Chem Bio CBR 4.0 water reservoir is one of the best water bladders available. This system can prevent the accidental swallowing of radioactive particulate when they need to take a drink.

It would also be a good idea to include swimmers' goggles so their eyes can be protected.

If your local school does not have a nuclear emergency protocol plan in place, reach out to the principal and help them to develop one. Nuclear emergencies are no longer hypothetical situations. They are real-life emergencies that we cannot afford to ignore.

Give their teacher and/or the principal of your school the contact numbers for your relatives and friends that could pick up your child if you could not reach the area. Give your child a card with that information, laminate it or put it in a plastic bag and sew it into their backpack.

Understanding Radiation and Its Effects

To design a radiation protection or shelter plan for any type of nuclear emergency, you need to know how to measure exposure. Begin by learning the standard units of measurement: *rads, roentgens* and *rems.* Roentgens (R) measure the levels of gamma and X-radiation energy production per cubic centimeter of air. Rads (for "radiation absorbed dose") measure the amount of radiation absorbed by any given material, living bodies included. One roentgen of gamma radiation exposure is roughly equivalent to one rad of absorbed dose. Rems measure absorbed radiation levels in humans specifically. Rems is the measurement expressed by "R" in the material below. Dose rate meters and dosimeters measure radiation exposure levels by Roentgens (R), Milliroentgens (mR), Gray's (Gr) or Sievert's (Sy).

Different materials exposed to equal levels of radiation absorb different amounts. For example, the chitin exoskeleton of a cockroach allows it to scurry away from radiation that would quickly kill a human. Chitin is a more difficult material for the radioactive energy to penetrate than human skin. The following chart, taken from the NATO's and other handbooks on nuclear event health and safety, outlines radiation's health effects. The figures assume that the cumulative total radiation exposure was all received within one week.

Total Exposure, Onset and Duration of Initial Symptoms:

- 30 to 70 R…From 6–12 hours: none to slight incidence of transient headache and nausea; vomiting in up to 5% of personnel in upper part of dose range; lymphocyte depression within 24 hours. Full recovery expected.
- 70 to 150 R…From 2–20 hours: transient mild nausea and vomiting in 5%–30%; potential for delayed traumatic and surgical wound healing; minimal clinical effect. Moderate drop in lymphocyte, platelet, and granulocyte counts. Increased susceptibility to opportunistic pathogens. Full recovery expected.
- 150 to 300 **R**…From 2 hours to 3 days: transient to moderate nausea and vomiting in 20%–70%; mild to moderate fatigability and weakness in 25%–60%. At 3 to 5 weeks: medical care required for 10%–50%. At high end of range, 10% may die. Anticipated medical problems include infection, bleeding, and fever. Wounds and burns geometrically increase morbidity and mortality.
- 300 to 530 R…From 2 hours to 3 days: transient to moderate nausea and vomiting and mild to moderate fatigability in 50%–90%. At 2 to 5 weeks: medical care required for 10%–80%. At low end of range, fewer than 10% deaths; at high end, death may occur for more than 50%. Anticipated medical problems include frequent diarrhea, anorexia, increased fluid loss, and ulceration. Increased infection susceptibility during immunocompromised time frame. Moderate to severe loss of lymphocytes. Hair loss after 14 days.
- 530 to 830 R…From 2 hours to 2 days: moderate to severe nausea and vomiting in 80%–100%; from 2 hours to 6 weeks: moderate to severe fatigability and weakness in 90%–100% of personnel. At 10 days to 5 weeks: medical care required for 50%–100%. At low end of range, death may occur for more than 50% at six weeks. At high end, death may occur for 99%. Anticipated medical problems include developing pathogenic and opportunistic infections, bleeding, fever, loss of appetite, ulcerations, bloody diarrhea, severe fluid and electrolyte shifts, capillary leak, hypotension. Combined with any significant physical trauma, survival rates will approach zero.
- 830 R or more…From 30 minutes to 2 days: severe nausea, vomiting, fatigability, weakness, dizziness, and disorientation; moderate to severe fluid imbalance and headache. Total bone marrow depletion within days. CNS symptoms are predominant at higher radiation levels. Few, if any, survivors even with aggressive and immediate medical attention.

Some people have a high radiation tolerance, others, low. To be safe, assume yours is low. The body responds better to radiation exposure extended over a long time than to one highly concentrated dose, so you should remove yourself quickly from an area contaminated with radioactive material. The faster you get away, the smaller the cumulative dose.

Potassium Iodide and Potassium Iodate

Potassium iodide and potassium iodate pills can block thyroidal absorption of radioiodine, a radioisotopic product of nuclear explosions and nuclear power plant accidents. Potassium iodate has an extra oxygen atom said to extend its shelf life and to make it taste better. It is also easier for children to use because of the neutral taste and smaller dosage. Most KI-KIO3 tablets are 85mg and only need to be taken once a day. Before adding these to your nuclear event survival supplies, check with your doctor. They may be dangerous for some people, including those with the following medical conditions: hyperthyroidism (thyrotoxicosis), Graves' disease, thyroid carcinoma, subacute thyroiditis, Hashimoto's thyroiditis, adenomas, McCune-Albright syndrome, excessive TSH secretion, iodized table salt allergy, hypocomplementaemic vasculitis, certain kidney and adrenal problems, and dermatitis herpetiformis. They may also be unsafe for those taking hypertension medication, quinidine, enalopril, or captopril. Follow the different dosage instructions for adults and children carefully.

When To Take KI or KIO3:

Hopefully, the local authorities will eventually notify you of a radiation hazard over the radio or television. If they don't, a Nukalert radiation alarm, dosimeter or dose rate meter will clue you in for certainty's sake about these hazards.

IA TIP

Before swallowing ipecac syrup to induce vomiting, *e.g.,* after an accidental potassium iodate overdose, take a small quantity of Pepto-Bismol. This will help to coat and protect the esophagus.

Emergency Shelters from Nuclear Emergencies

If you own a home, you may want to consider purchasing an emergency shelter. The modern ones offer much more protection than their 1950s counterparts.

The best civilian nuclear emergency shelters available today are sold by Radius Engineering, Inc. and designed by Walton McCarthy, a member of the American Society of Mechanical Engineers and the technical advisory board for the American Civil Defense Association. His research into nuclear shelter design began in 1978 and led to the engineering bible for nuclear shelters, *Principles of Nuclear Protection*. Shelters based on his designs vary in size to hold different numbers of persons and are self-contained, with a three-stage air filtration system, leaching septic tank, deep-cycle batteries for lights and electronic equipment, and a separate underground generator.

These shelters can also be used during earthquakes, floods, tornadoes, and other emergencies.

It is important to learn what you can about nuclear emergencies and their effects. I suggest that you read *Nuclear War Survival Skills* by Cresson H. Kearny, which is considered the bible of nuclear emergency information. You can download it for free at www.oism.org/nwss or www.ki4u.com/free_book. Shane Conner of KI4U.com has also assembled useful information on his website www.ki4u.com/survive/doomsday.htm. As Shane said to me in a recent conversation, there is "good news," that if you survive the initial blast, there is no reason why you cannot avoid and survive the horrific aftereffects.

CHAPTER 23

Crime Prevention
for the Home

PREPAREDNESS FOR HUMAN-MADE EMERGENCIES AND NATURAL DISASTERS IS A CONCERTED to maintain control of our lives and the means to protect loved ones. It seems almost instinctive to want to secure one's home; this chapter attempts to address ways of doing so without spending a fortune in the process.

To take practical countermeasures against crime one must first understand the standard operating procedure of criminals.

The most powerful thing one can do to protect against burglary is to increase the difficulty of entry. Increasing the time a criminal must spend trying to enter both discourages the burglar and makes it easier for cops or a frightened homeowner to apprehend him. The best way to do this is to:

- Secure all the points of entry. Strong window gates with quick-release levers or locks discourage the average thief and can be quickly removed in case of fire.
- Add multiple locks that are difficult to pick or force open to all of the doors. Don't forget that a security door is only as strong as its frame— make sure yours is in decent shape, or replace it.
- Never leave keys under mats, rugs, lights, or any place where you think burglars won't look. (They will.)
- Keep the outer areas to your home well lit. Most burglars act under the cover of darkness and are discouraged from working in an illuminated area. If your situation allows it, install solar-powered emergency lights to save money and keep your home safer during power outages, which tend to encourage burglars and even more dangerous predators. Light all possible points of entry. Also get rid of any shrubbery or other inessential growth or structures near your home that burglars could hide behind while they work.
- Keep curtains or blinds closed. Don't give strangers the opportunity to know what you own or good views of your house. If a burglar casing for an easy mark can spot your 70-inch HDTV and costly laptop through your living room window, he might become inspired to attempt a break-in.

A burglar hot enough for your shiny toys might attempt a push-and-enter, knocking at your door. If you fall for his ruse, he can use the element of surprise to knock you off balance and force his way inside. Push-and-enter thieves tend to be high, armed and as violent and crazy as they are greedy. Burglars and other criminals can spy you from the street, from inside your apartment building, or even from a nearby home. If your neighbor has unsavory friends, they might be monitoring your daily routine from the neighbor's apartment. Some will even try to befriend you, to gain access to your home so they can case it from the inside. Love your neighbors. Just don't trust them unless you know them well.

For electronic home security systems, I like using a combination of cleverly hidden and strategically placed motion sensors with loud alarms, along with video surveillance cameras with infrared capabilities. The motion sensors can alert you to suspicious movement within your home, while infrared video cameras can provide images even when it is dark. Some special cameras can be connected to your computer and allow you to keep watch on your home even when at work or on vacation. Veo Observer makes a great camera with a built-in server that allows the cameras to stream images and audio over the Internet without routing them through a PC. They can pan and tilt to give you a wider viewing area than fixed cameras.

Quad manufactures an indoor/outdoor home video surveillance system with an infrared-enabled camera, motion detector, audio pickup, and intercom that lets you speak to an intruder. It is small enough to be hidden, is simple to set up, and operates with up to four cameras. Place the monitors in secure areas of your home (such as your bedroom) where you can safely watch an intruder and phone for help.

Motion sensors outdoors, and indoors if you have pets, must be "pet immune," *i.e.*, able to distinguish pets and small wild animals from human beings. This prevents false alarms.

Presence sensors can be mounted near your front or back door, steps, or anywhere with flooring or deck material where someone would stand. They are activated by pressure, are weather-hardy, and not triggered by pets.

Basic combinations of these devices allow you to detect and, if you choose, intercept anyone who enters or gets too near your home. A drawback of all of them is that they cannot operate during power outages unless you have an emergency power supply. If you're handy, you can make a low-tech but highly effective noisemaker burglar alarm. You need some monofilament fishing line, eyelet screws, and a blank shotgun shell.

This type of trip alarm can be easily mounted near any entrance. The alarm is set off by pressure applied to the trip wire threaded through the eyelets and tightened near a door, window, or any other portal into your home. The pressure releases the firing pin, setting off a 12-gauge blank cartridge. The loud shotgun blast will alert you and probably scare the intruder away. Handle the blanks with care—they can do a lot of damage if mishandled!

If the sound of a shotgun shell firing doesn't discourage the intruder, a blast from a pepper gas dispenser will. DefenseDevices.com sells a pepper spray booby trap that releases four ounces of pepper gas, quickly filling the surrounding air with incapacitating fumes once a wire is tripped. Most burglars are unprepared for this painful surprise. The noxious fumes will motivate most thieves to make a quick exit. After released, the pepper-spray will not stain or linger on your furniture. The canisters are replaceable and easily installed along with the dispensers. If you decide to use a pepper spray dispenser, have a plan and the means of protecting yourself from the fumes should it ever be triggered, such as a 3M R-95 respirator.

Beware of fake UPS or FedEx delivery persons. Like those of police officers and firefighters, a UPS or FedEx uniform is almost a free entry pass for a thief or worse. Ask a UPS or FedEx delivery person to show you his or her ID, so you will be able to distinguish them from fakes.

Thieves know that people trust doormen and security guards by sight. Don't let a blue uniform trick you into a false sense of security. For many security companies, the most stringent requirement for employment is to be able to fit the suit.

Even seeming police officers should be checked out before they're allowed into your home. Authentic badges and uniforms are available online and from many stores across the country. When someone who appears to be a police officer asks to cross your door, politely ask why he or she is there and evaluate the response carefully. Before you open your door, ask him or her to stand in front of your peephole so that you can see the badge number, then ask him or her to recite it. Ask the officer to specify his or her precinct; inspect uniforms and behavior for irregularities. Police cannot enter your home without a search warrant unless they have reason to believe that a dangerous situation necessitates their intervention. If they have a warrant, ask to see it. Ignore your rights at your peril.

Your home security plan should cover peripheral areas. Establish a post office box and have all of your important mail delivered there if the mailbox at your home is not secure. If you live in an apartment building with a basement laundry room, remember that washing machines and dryers produce a white noise that can mask cries for help. Wash your clothes while the area has some traffic, and encourage your landlord to install security cameras. If you park in a building with a large garage, listen for footsteps, look underneath vehicles for feet, and keep an eye and ear out for unfamiliar faces or suspicious activity.

Never take out the trash at night unless your garbage collection area is well lit and in view of passers-by. Try to keep your pepper spray or other weapon in your hand when you travel to areas peripheral to your home.

Some of these measures may seem extreme, but the increased sophistication of criminal take advantage of the easygoing and unskeptical. Become more observant, become more secure.

CHAPTER 24

The 21st-Century Home

"Our house was our castle and our keep
Our house in the middle of our street
Our house that was where we used to sleep
Our house in the middle of our street"

—Madness

YOUR HOME SHOULD BE A STURDY CASTLE THAT CAN PROVIDE YOU WITH PROTECTION FROM many of the troubles mentioned throughout this book, including the less sexy problem of indoor air pollution. Even if you live in an apartment, dramatic changes can be made that will help you to build a safer and healthier home.

If you are thinking about building a new home, the purpose of this chapter is to show you some non-traditional designs for homes that are many times more energy-efficient than traditional structures. Twenty-first-century homes should be disaster-resistant, low-maintenance, and energy independent. I consider it one of my missions to convince readers to leave their old tinderboxes behind for good.

The last important lesson in this chapter is for those who want to disconnect from the grid and build a homestead. The last section will show you how to get started.

Eliminating Indoor Air Pollution

The EPA considers indoor air pollution to be one of the most serious environmental hazards of the new century. Their studies and publications (*Indoor Air Pollution: An Introduction for Health Professionals*) have concluded that air inside many American homes could be from 100 to 400 times more polluted than the air in Los Angeles. The ACA (American College of Allergists) states that 50% of all illnesses are aggravated or caused by indoor air pollution. These appalling facts have forced the American Lung association to declare that as of 2005, three out of five people suffer respiratory and breathing problems.

Some of the nastiest indoor air pollution originates from household cleaning sprays, paints, air fresheners, polishes, disinfectants, solvents, adhesives, insecticides, and other frequently used chemicals. Even cheap furniture made out of particleboard, plywood, certain types of paneling, and synthetic fabrics give off toxic fumes.

Some companies proudly proclaim that their cleaning product can kill 99.5% of all microorganisms in your bathroom and kitchen. But you are also an organism, and the germicidal chemicals in these cleaners can also damage your health—and that of your children, born or unborn. These chemicals combine with the effluvia of synthetic fabrics, cheap furniture, pesticides, cosmetics (hair spray, deodorant, perfumes), and dry-cleaned clothing. This toxic mix enters our bodies through our skin, inhalation, and ingestion, producing respiratory illness, memory loss, headaches, allergies, and central nervous system problems. In some extreme cases, prolonged exposure can damage the liver and kidneys and even cause cancer.

Another cause of the increase in interior air pollution is over-insulation. Our efforts at energy conservation have driven us to build hyper-insulated homes that seal us indoors tighter than a submarine. Without proper ventilation, all the insulation helps produce a "sick house syndrome" in which indoor air pollution can cause physical discomfort, even illness.

Air pollution indoors is exacerbated by outdoor air pollution, especially for those who live in large cities or near industrial areas. Contaminants outside your home combine with the indoor pollutants, magnifying their impact on your health.

Over the next two decades, population increases will likely produce further congestion, waste, energy consumption, and, probably, more outdoor and indoor air pollution. Small towns are not pollution-free: tiny airborne particles, ozone, lead, and other contaminants are making the air unfit to breathe everywhere. In 2000, the *New England Journal of Medicine* reported that these substances are causing large numbers of illnesses and even deaths among the elderly and people with respiratory problems.

You may not be able to control the air quality on the outside, but you certainly can on the inside of your home if you take the following steps:

Eliminate Toxic Household Products:

Start with insecticides, carpet-, oven-, furniture-, glass-, and bathroom-cleaners, and polishes that contain toxic chemicals such as ammonia and chlorine. Many highly effective, nonpolluting insecticides and household cleaners are now available. Some may be more costly, but your lungs will thank you. The following are some of the best:

Household All-Purpose Cleaners:

First Generation Soap and Clothing Detergent, Citra-Solv, Dr. Bronner's Castile Soap, Ajax Lemon Fresh Liquid (diluted 1:50), EarthRite, Crocodile Clean, Best Darn Soap, Ecover, Envirrone, Mr. Clean, Murphy's Oil Soap, and Spic and Span.

Oven Cleaners:

Try regular soap and a steel wool pad. This will not only do the trick, but also give you a little workout in the process.

Bathroom and Kitchen Cleaners:

You don't need to purchase toxic bathroom disinfectants that poison the environment after being flushed down the sink and toilet. A Virginia Polytechnic Institute food scientist, Susan Sumner, created a simple formula for a strong disinfecting spray. All you need to make it is hydrogen peroxide (3% solution) and white or apple cider vinegar, and a pair of spray bottles. When you clean your kitchen counter, vegetables, or even toilet, spray them with the vinegar and hydrogen peroxide solutions in either order. Thoroughly rinse the vegetables or surface with water. In laboratory tests, the combined mists killed practically all *E. coli,* salmonella, and shigella bacteria on contaminated food and hard surfaces. This simple spray combination was more effective at killing dangerous bacteria than chlorine bleach or any regular kitchen cleaning solution. Spray them separately—don't mix them.

Identify, Control, and Eliminate Other Sources of Interior Air Pollution:

Among the worst offenders are poorly maintained vacuum cleaners, fireplaces, and furnaces. Vacuum cleaner filters must be regularly changed to insure clean operation (HEPA filters are best). Fireplaces and furnaces must be meticulously maintained for optimal operation. You should learn as much as you can about cleaning and servicing your furnace. If not, be prepared to pay professional cleaners a tidy sum for a task that is simple enough to complete yourself.

Washing machines are also major sources of indoor air pollution. When placed in improperly ventilated areas, they release harmful contaminants into the air during chemical volatilization, when the agitation, heat, and other conditions inside the machine strip away harmful chemicals such as ethanol (from detergent) and chlorine (bleach) and deposit them into the surrounding air.

Carpets trap dirt, dust, pollen and other irritants that can aggravate allergies and other more serious respiratory conditions such as asthma. Plastics and other synthetic or chemically treated fabric and other materials such as particleboard, plywood, and CCA (chromium, copper, and arsenic-treated wood) release highly toxic fumes into the air through outgassing.

Radon gas is another form of indoor air pollution, and one of the most dangerous. This radioactive gas is, next to smoking, the leading cause of lung cancer. One in 15 American homes has high radon levels. Radon comes from rock, earth, building materials, and in some cases well water. Homes should be tested by a professional for radon gas to ensure their safety. The EPA can provide you with information about testing.

Mold is one of the most difficult sources of indoor air pollution to control or eliminate. It is very hardy and can grow on many different types of household surfaces. When spores enter your home, they settle on damp spots, feeding on whatever is available on the surface. Some mold produces airborne mycotoxins that can sicken or, in high concentrations, kill. It is practically impossible to eliminate mold, but it can be controlled by reducing the moisture levels in the air and meticulous housecleaning, especially on surfaces that are exposed to water, such as bathroom tiles. Check your home for leaky pipes and moisture spots. When you find them, call a professional to make the proper repairs (unless you can do them yourself), and thoroughly clean the surrounding area.

Vapor condensation is another cause of mold growth. You can help eliminate it by improving ventilation in areas where moisture tends to build up, such as the kitchen and bathroom. Vapor barriers, dehumidifiers, insulated storm windows, and doors will also help. If possible, substitute area rugs for wall-to-wall carpets. If you already have carpet in place, make sure to wash it regularly. It's also good to have people remove their shoes at the entryway. To monitor your moisture problem, buy a hygrometer at your local hardware store and install it near the trouble spots.

In the summertime, **clean air conditioner vents** and drip pans frequently, especially after heavy use. Check all of your ventilation and heating ducts for mold. Make sure to wear a particulate respirator (N-95 to N-100 rating) over your face along with a hair cover and gloves. If you can't see anything and want to be sure that none is present, buy a mold testing kit from a good hardware store or on the Internet. If you find mold, contact professional duct cleaning contractors to have it removed.

Insects, certain types of plants, and animals can also produce irritating particulate material that can cause health problems, especially for people with respiratory problems and allergies. Dead skin flakes (dander) from cats and dogs—and other mammals that people now keep as pets—can mix with other airborne particles such as dried and pulverized insect body parts and feces, pollen, and dust. If you own pets, keep them as clean as possible. If you have carpets or rugs, clean them frequently and thoroughly in every area of your home where animals spend time. Insects can be controlled by removing garbage, papers, or cardboard boxes and other objects that they tend to hide inside and lay their eggs. Regularly clean areas where insects tend to live, use natural pesticides to kill them, and keep food stored in airtight containers.

Smokers produce severe indoor air pollution problems that can only be remedied by their quitting, or by their being restricted to areas with a separate ventilation system. Smoking in your home deposits toxic contents of cigarette smoke into your furniture and every other porous thing, including you.

Increase Ventilation:

Good ventilation can help reduce interior air pollution if you live where the outside air is relatively clean. To keep interior air pollution levels low and the air fresh, the air in your home should be exchanged every three to four hours. Keeping your windows open or installing ventilation fans is more than enough to get the job done. If you live in a large city near congested roads, highways, garbage-filled streets, or a large industrial area, this may not be wise.

Buy Air Filtration Devices and/or Houseplants:

If you can afford it, buy air filtration devices. If you can't, certain types of houseplants can do the trick. Plants are living air filters that not only beautify your environment, but also absorb and eliminate many pollutants in the same way as high-tech electronic devices. According to Dr. Bill Wolverton, a former NASA scientist and author of *Eco-Friendly Houseplants,* some of the best are the lady palm, golden pothos, areca palm, and *ficus alii.* Three large plants per 100 square feet should do the trick for an average apartment.

A good air cleaner can help minimize and in some cases practically eliminate harmful substances from the air. One of the best air cleaners is called an **air ionizer**. The U.S. Dept. of Agriculture found that using an ionizer in a regular-sized room removed more than half of the suspended dust particles, and nearly all the bacteria. Many of the pollutants found in the air ride on floating dust particles.

If you put an ionizer in each room in your living space, they will make a tremendous difference in your air quality. If your home has a carpet, ionizers help to reduce a large amount of the materials released into the air when you walk. Always place them in an elevated location near a fan or air supply vent so that the negative ions can be optimally distributed. In large rooms, move them toward the center. If you suffer from allergies or other respiratory problems, the unit should be close to where you sit, work, or stand.

Most good ionizers discharge high-voltage electrical current up small slivers of metal "needlepoints" to generate the negative ions. Check for the units with the most needlepoints. They should also be made out of stainless steel for durability and easy to clean. Expect to spend about $70 dollars per unit—a relatively small price to pay for improving your air quality and health.

HEPA Filters:

HEPA (High Efficiency Particulate Air) filters are the best type available for removing small particles from the air. The operational standards for all HEPA filters state that they must capture a minimum of 99.97% of contaminants larger than 0.3 microns.

HEPA filters are used in many environments, including hospitals, high-tech equipment manufacturing, and the pharmaceutical industry. In open environments, I prefer houseplants or ionizers, because they tend to draw suspended particles out of the air instead of sucking them into a machine. It is not a very efficient way of cleaning your air, unless the filter is attached to a sealed device such as an air blower or a vacuum cleaner. They can also be more expensive.

HEPA filters work well as central units attached to ventilation systems or in small poorly ventilated areas. They are also great for cars, especially for commuters who spend much time in traffic. Most portable HEPA units come with jacks that can be plugged directly into the dashboard for ease of use.

Keeping the air clean in your home, vehicle, office or any other space where you spend the bulk of your time should be one of your top priorities. The long-term benefits to your health far outweigh any expense and work involved in setup.

Alternative Homebuilding

Non-traditional alternative home designs offer so many benefits, that traditional homes pale in comparison. They are much more energy-efficient, environmentally friendly, fire- and termite-proof, disaster-resistant, and many can last for centuries. They can easily absorb the impact of hurricanes. Katrina and Rita would have blown right past them.

Earthquakes hardly leave a crack, and some have actually been tested in and survived simulated nuclear explosions.

You might feel that a home of this type is financially beyond your reach. It probably isn't. Some can cost considerably less than a traditional home. Others cost about the same to build as a regular structure. Another added benefit is that most alternative homes can be constructed in less than half the time of a regular home. When you take all these facts into consideration, why would you build anything else?

The first and most popular alternative home design was invented over 60 years ago by the late great design scientist/architect/philosopher R. Buckminster Fuller. He created the Geodome to provide the world with inexpensive disaster-resistant shelter that was simple to construct, transport and environmentally friendly.

Geodomes are not just for emergency shelter, as you read in Chapter 8—they also make the perfect 21st-century home. I believe that the time has come for us to fully capitalize on Dr. Fuller's wonderful contribution to the world and make Geodesic Dome homes the standard by which all other homes are measured.

Geodomes use an arrangement of triangles fashioned roughly into the shape of a hemisphere. The structural elements equally divide the total load of the structure, giving the dome exceptional strength and durability.

Geodomes also have more space than a traditional structure, because their semispherical configuration has the highest ratio of enclosed area to external surface area of any shape. A carbon atom cluster discov-

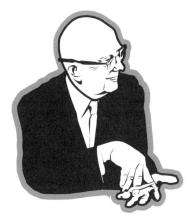

Buckminster Fuller

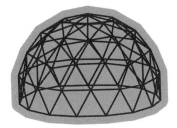

Geodome

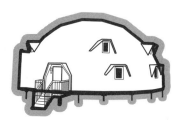

American Ingenuity Dome

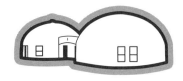

Monolithic Domes

ered in the early 1990s of the same design was named by scientists the "Buckminsterfullerine."

Geodomes are far more durable, use much less material, and are easier to build than their old-world counterparts. Best of all, they require half the energy required to heat or cool as an old-style structure. Most new Geodome home packages cost less than half of a comparable sized traditional home—and much less if you are willing to do some of the work yourself.

Several companies offer Geodomes, but American Ingenuity (www. aidomes.com) manufactures a prefabricated, steel-reinforced concrete Geodesic dome home kit that is easy to build, inexpensive, disaster-resistant, completely fireproof, and beautiful. American Ingenuity Geodesic dome homes can withstand a direct hit by a large hurricane and even some tornadoes. A termite would break his mandibles on them, and they don't need roofing.

Another company called Monolithic Domes Inc. (www.monolithic.com) located in Texas specializes in steel-reinforced domes with thin concrete shells that are even more disaster-resistant and durable. They are more expensive than American Ingenuity domes, but worth it.

Formworks Building Company (www.formworksbuilding.com) offers the most disaster-resistant structures outside of storm shelters. They are high-quality thin-shell concrete domes called Nest Egg Homes, and are designed to be earth-covered. Nest Egg homes need no external maintenance, and are highly tornado-, hurricane- and earthquake-resistant. These are the homes I mentioned earlier that could withstand earthquakes (7.1 with no damage) and simulated nuclear explosions. They cost more than the Monolithic or Geodomes to build, but no more than a regular wood frame home. The extraordinary benefits that you receive far outweigh the additional expenses. The money saved from heating and maintenance alone will eventually pay for the extra cost.

Quite simply, these structures are the wave of the future. Old-style wood frame homes should now be considered obsolete. They are expensive and slow to construct, waste energy, consume enormous amounts of timber (100 large trees per home) and are flimsy compared to their Geodesic counterparts. We should finally say goodbye to these 18th-century relics once and for all.

You might want to add a renewable energy solar, wind or even a hydrogen fuel cell power system to make your geodesic dome home into an energy-independent, off-grid 21st-century rural homestead. If you do, you will need to know the following:

Where do you plan to build your home?
It is recommended that you build your home on high ground, away from rivers, lakes and oceans to avoid large-scale floods. If you plan to use the land to

grow food, you will need to find a location with nutrient-rich soil that can support growth.

Does your property have a water supply?

If it doesn't have a well or spring, you will need to connect to your local source. If not, you must purchase cisterns to collect rainwater, and pumps, filters and water tanks to keep it stored away and potable.

What about travel? How close will your home be to a highway or road?

If you do not have a reliable form of transportation, you should keep it as accessible as possible.

Do you have homebuilding skills?

If you don't, you are at a disadvantage because you will be dependent on contractors to build your home. This can significantly drive up the cost.

Sanitation?

The best sanitation systems for this type of home are composting toilets. They are simple, easy to maintain and inexpensive. Septic systems are complex, costly and difficult to install and maintain.

Personal safety?

Even a rural homestead can see criminal activity. You must be prepared to encounter it if and when it comes.

Tools and equipment?

You will likely need tools for construction, plumbing, carpentry, gardening, masonry, and metalwork, and precision tools for electrical work.

Electrical energy needs?

You must know what it will be so you can purchase a renewable energy system that can meet your demands. To make an accurate calculation, add up the load (amount of electrical energy used) of every single electrical device that you will be using. Remember, some devices have variable loads such as blenders, microwaves, washing machines, dishwashers. etc.

IA TIP

Renewable-energy power system owners know that it is best to eliminate as many non-essential electrical devices and appliances as possible. Make sure to use energy-efficient lights, appliances, fans, stereos, etc. Base your calculations of total load on every single device operating at their maximum capacity, and simultaneously.

How much energy (in watts) does each appliance or device use? How many hours a day do you regularly operate them? Multiply the watts × hours of usage. Add 30% to your total to allow for system losses. Your total is the amount of energy that each appliance uses in watt-hours.

Once you have an accurate number, you can begin to search for a high-quality renewable energy system package that corresponds with your needs. If you live in a "solar friendly" area like Arizona, New Mexico or Florida you can go completely solar. In a state with more temperate weather, you may need to use what is called a hybrid renewable energy power system. This is simply a combination of different types of renewable energy generators working together like a wrestling tag team. When one fails to generate sufficient power, the other kicks in and takes up the slack. Hybrid systems are usually comprised of solar panels and wind turbines, the occasional micro-hydroelectric systems and diesel generators as a back-up.

Residential hydrogen fuel cells are just hitting the market and even more exotic generators like Stirling engines are now available. These are heat-powered motors that use expanding gas to move a magnet through a coil to generate electrical current. A company called Whisper Gen (www.whispergen.com) manufactures a Stirling Motor that can be used as a residential power unit.

To get started on learning more about renewable energy, consult the following books:

- *The Complete Idiot's Guide to Solar Power for Your Home* by Dan Ramsey
- *The Solar Electric House: Energy for the Environmentally Responsive, Energy-Independent Home* by Stephen Strong
- *Wind Energy Basics* by Paul Gipe
- *Wind Power Workshop* by Hugh Piggott
- *Real Goods Solar Living Sourcebook* by John Schaffer

If you make the wise decision to build one of the suggested homes and move inside, you might wonder how you ever managed to live without one. The 21st-Century Home closes the circle of this life-defense program.

One last thing…

The best form of emergency preparedness is to support organizations and individuals who struggle to improve the conditions on our interstellar oasis. They need all the help that they can get. Anything that you can do to help makes a difference.

Greenpeace USA
702 H Street NW, Suite 300
Washington, DC 20001
www.greenpeace.org/usa

Unicef
Call 1.800.4UNICEF to make a donation by phone.
To make a donation by mail, send with a check or money order payable to the U.S. Fund for UNICEF to:

www.unicefusa.org
333 East 38th Street
New York, NY 10016

Care
Make a credit card donation by calling:
800-521-CARE ext. 999
www.careusa.org

Doctors Without Borders
333 7th Avenue, 2nd Floor
New York, NY 10001
www.doctorswithoutborders.org

Habitat For Humanity
121 Habitat Street
Americus, GA 31709-3498
www.habitat.org

Sierra Club
85 Second Street, 2nd Floor
San Francisco, CA 94105
information@sierraclub.org
www.sierraclub.org

Riverkeeper
mail checks to Riverkeeper Inc.
828 Broadway
Tarrytown, NY 10591
www.riverkeeper.org

Preparedness Source List

Emergency Evacuation Cards are available to download
and print at **www.PreparednessNow.net**

EMERGENCY EVACUATION CARD

Notes

Alternate Locations

EMERGENCY EVACUATION CARD

Address 1 _____ Start _____AM _____AM
                                                       PM   PM
_____ Frequency _____

_____ Days _____

Address 2 _____ Start _____AM _____AM
                                                       PM   PM
_____ Frequency _____

_____ Days _____

Locations _____

_____

Emergency Telephone Numbers _____

_____

HERE ARE MY FAVORITE SOURCES FOR EMERGENCY PREPAREDNESS-RELATED EQUIPMENT including some of the harder-to-find items listed in this book.

One-Stop Preparedness Shopping

Most goods needed for E-Kits, Grab-and-Go Bags, food, first aid, sanitation, shelter, lighting, power, heating, emergency communication and self-defense can all be found from one vendor, making their acquisition a simpler task.

Nitro-Pak Preparedness Center
800.866.4876   fax: 888.648.7672
www.nitro-pak.com
Nitro-Pak is the largest mail-order company in the country that specializes in emergency preparedness supplies and freeze-dried food.

Major Surplus and Survival
800.441.8855   fax: 310.324.6909
www.majorsurplusnsurvival.com
Major Surplus and Survival is a good source for hard-to-find items that can enhance your total preparedness package.

EMS (Eastern Mountain Sports)
888.463.6367
www.ems.com
EMS is one of my favorite sources for stoves, tents, rappelling equipment and other types of camping supplies. The employees are knowledgeable and friendly.

Cabela's
800.237.4444
www.cabelas.com

Ready Me
(310) 398-5700
www.ready-me.com
Ready Me grab and go bags and emergency kits are all top grade. They are designed for real-world situations and do not contain any 'filler' items. All of the components are extremely durable and of the highest quality. Ready Me bags are the only pre-prepared types that I would personally recommend and use.

One Stop "Mil-Spec" Gear

The following outlets specialize in clothing and gear for police and military who already need to keep preparedness in mind. Items for E-Kits, Grab-and-Go Bags, self-defense, food, personal protective equipment, sanitation and emergency communication are available from the merchants below.

Brigade Quartermasters
800.388.4327
www.actiongear.com
Brigade Quartermasters is the place to go for equipment manufactured to military specifications and also for important preparedness items.

Tad Gear, Inc.
415.318.8252
www.tadgear.com
Tad Gear carries top-quality products used by military personnel and serious outdoorsmen and women.

U.S. Cavalry
800.777.7172 fax: 270.352.0266
www.uscav.com
A good source of mil-spec equipment.

Shomer-Tec
www.shomer-tec.com
Shomer-Tec carries hard-to-find self-defense items.

Ranger Joe's Military and Law Enforcement Gear
800.247.4541
www.rangerjoe.com
More mil-spec items.

Cheaper Than Dirt
800.559.0943
www.cheaperthandirt.com
A mix of camping supplies and shooting sports gear.

E-Kit Pouches

Your E-Kit items, as described in Chapter 3, need to be held in a secure way attached to your person. Here are your best options.

Civilian Lab
www.civilianlab.com
626.744.0662
I recommend Civilian Lab's Covert Harness Bags as the best choice for an E-Kit Pouch. They can be worn discreetly, breathe well and carry a lot of gear.

Nite-Ize
www.niteize.com
Pock-Its are sold by many hardware and camping stores. The Mini Pock-Its and Hip Pock-Its hang less discreetly from your belt, but hold a good amount of E-Kit items securely.

Grab-and-Go Bags
How to carry the items described in Chapter 4.

Eagle Gear
800.695.3245 fax: 530.221.3506
www.eaglegear.com
I use the Eagle War Bag as my own Grab-and-Go Bag.

Battery-Free Flashlights and Radios

You'll want to have these in your Grab-and-Go Bag, also in your home and car.

Applied Innovative Technologies, Inc.
303.857.1405
www.appliedinnotech.com
Makes NightStar shake-to-recharge flashlights.

Freeplay
www.freeplayenergy.com
Freeplay makes the Free Charge Weza step treadle to jump start a car, cellphone or other battery-dependent things. Freeplay is an inventive leader in non-battery technology for emergency radios and flashlights.

Lentek Dynamo Torch
407.857.8786
www.lentek.com

Battery-Powered Flashlights

You'll need a powerful mini-flashlight for your E-Kit and other non-incendive varieties to supplement the shake or wind-up non-battery versions for the power of their beam. Remember to stock up on extra batteries for your homestead.

Product Wizard
www.productwizard.com
Carries all sorts of flashlights, including: Inova X5, Microlight, 24-7, X-1, X0, X03

Streamlight
www.streamlight.com
Manufactures and sells industrial-quality flashlights.

Water Purification

For inside and outside the home. See Chapters 4 and 7 for further information.

Katadyn
800.755.6701
www.katadyn.com
Excellent lightweight devices that purify questionable water sources on camping trips or during emergencies. Available from Brigade Quartermasters and other camping websites and stores.

British Berkefeld Water Filtration Systems
888.803.4438
www.newmillconcepts.com
The website above is for the American distributor of what I believe is the best home water filtration system.

Epets.com
Sells automatic food and water dispensers for your pet.

Emergency Cooking/Heating

See Chapters 4 and 7 for further information.

Four Dog Stove
763.444.9587
www.fourdog.com
Fine handcrafted stoves that can be used for emergency heating and cooking in the field and at home.

ZZ Manufacturing, Inc.
www.zzstove.com
The lightweight and reliable Sierra Stove uses charcoal, twigs, pinecones, shredded paper and other solid fuels to produce its flame. Its battery-powered fan can generate over 18,000 BTU/hr; enough heat to boil a quart of water in four minutes.

Solar Chargers

You should have a solar charger in your Grab-and-Go Bag. Batteries at times become too heavy, cumbersome and rare. See Chapters 4 and 10 for further information.

Sundance Solar
www.sundancesolar.com
Has Power Film solar battery chargers.

Solar Power Universal
www.onlybatteries.com

Self-Defense Products

To protect yourself and your family from two and four-legged beasts in frantic times. See Chapter 5: Self-Defense.

Shomer-Tec Inc
www.shomer-tec.com

TBO Tech
www.tbotech.com

Pepper Spray Training
The Center for Self-Preservation Training
Fight Fire With Fire video and manual.
www.demibarbito.com

The Survival Staff
www.crawfordknives.com
Handmade metal staff with blade in its interior. A good survival tool.

Smoke Escape Hoods/Gas Masks/Respirators

For more information on these items, see Chapter 6: Personal Protective Equipment.

Aramsco, Inc.
800.767.6933   fax: 856.848.0802

Essex PB&R
618.659.9070
www.smokehoods.com
Makes the Essex +10 Smoke Escape Hood.

National Institute for Occupational Safety and Health
800.35.NIOSH
www.cdc.gov/niosh/respinfo.html
Gas Mask Safety Information can be found here.

Phoenix
www.phoenixprotect.com

Safer America
866.SAFER.99
www.saferamerica.com
Safer America sells gas masks, even pet emergency respiratory equipment.

X-Caper Smoke Mask
888.777.7078
www.myxcaper.com

3M
www.3M.com
3M respirators are sold at most hardware and drug stores.

Water Storage

See Chapter 7: Water.

Aquatank
www.aquaflex.net

American Tanks Company
www.watertanks.com

Backpacks, Tents and Outdoor Gear

These manufacturers and merchants sell emergency shelters, outdoor gear and backpacks. These items are discussed in Chapter 10: Shelter.

Kelty
800.423.2320   fax: 800.504.2745
www.kelty.com
Kelty makes high-quality tents and backpacks.

The North Face
800.447.2333
www.thenorthface.com
North Face manufactures great winter clothing.

Coleman
800.835.3278
www.coleman.com
Coleman offers a large selection of preparedness-related items, including tents, backpacks, sleeping bags, flashlights, generators, lanterns, and inflatable boats.

Generators

See Chapters 10 and 24 for more information.

Home Depot
www.homedepot.com

Generator Joe
707.539.9003
www.generatorjoe.net
A one-stop source of information about all types of generators.

Northern Tool
www.northerntool.com

Sanitation Engineering

Read Chapter 11: Sanitation and Hygiene and the following books:
The Humanure Handbook by Joseph Jenkins
How to Shit in the Woods by Kathleen Mayer
(A great book to keep in your Grab-and-Go Bag.)

Emergency Transportation

Various options regarding getting away from disasters are discussed in Chapter 17.

Bicycles

Montague Corporation
800.736.5348
www.montagueco.com
www.civilianlab.com
The Montague folding bicycle is my choice of emergency transportation. It is lightweight, durable and reasonably priced. West Coasters can purchase them from Pasadena's Civilian Lab.

Dahon Bicycles
www.dahon.com
Dahon manufactures high quality and durable folding bikes.

Bicycle Tires, Airless

Air Free Tires, Inc.
800.771.9513
www.airfreetires.com

Air Filter Masks for Bicyclists

Greenscreen
www.mfiap.com/gs

Respro (UK) Ltd
www.respro.com

Mopeds, Scooters

www.mopedsonline.com

Solar Car Battery Charger

Real Goods
www.realgoods.com
You can also get a foot-crank FreeCharge Weza from Freeplay that can get the job done without waiting for a solar charge.
www.freeplayenergy.com

Wheelchair Bags

Medaid
800.743.7203
www.sportaid.com

Wheelsource
415.456.6134
www.wheelsource.com

Custom Mini-Pry Bars

You can always buy a $3 mini-pry bar from a local hardware store, but Peter Atwood's costly tools are designed to be easily carried and they perform flawlessly.

Peter Atwood
413.537.0472
www.phlaunt.com/atwoodknives

Fire Escape

For further information, see Chapter 19: Fire Prevention and Escape.

Fire Blankets

www.firesafetysource.com
877.520.9080

Fire Escape Ladders

Bold Industries
203.334.5237
www.boldindustries.com
The 50-ft. Res-Q-Ladder will get you out of the fifth or sixth floor of a building.

Emergency Parachutes

Aerial Egress, Inc.
909.940.1324
This is a last-resort option for people stuck in high-rise fires or accidents above 50 stories. Escape parachutes are risky, but the advantages may outweigh the drawbacks if you are ever caught in a high-rise with no other options.

Protective Clothing

Euclid Garment Mfg. Co.
330.673.7413
www.euclidgarment.com
This is industrial-grade haz-mat gear and footwear that might make you look like you belong in the band DEVO, but will protect you against chemical, biological and radiological difficulties. See Chapter 21: Chemical and Biological Warfare for further information.

Atropine Auto-Injectors

If you're particularly prepared, you'll have one of these to protect against Nerve Gas. Discussed in Chapter 21: Chemical and Biological Warfare.

Meridian Medical Technologies, Inc.
800.638.8093
government@meridianmt.com

Alternative Electrical Solutions

Solar Electricity

Here's a long-term solution to power grid instability. See Chapter 24: The 21st-Century Home for further information. I suggest that you subscribe to *Home Power* magazine, an invaluable resource regarding solar and renewable energy systems.
www.homepower.com

Real Goods
800.762.7325
www.realgoods.com
Excellent site for neophytes interested in learning about emergency solar power systems. Back in 1978, Real Goods primarily served rural homesteaders in what was once called the "back to the land" movement. Since then, they have strived to seek out environmentally-friendly technology for its customers. Their experience in renewable energy technology is extensive and they are willing to share it with all who are interested.

SolarSense.com
www.solarsense.com
Solarsense markets good emergency power systems, including a portable power pack called Nomad. The 300 unit can be used to power small devices. The 1500 unit can power up larger appliances.

Kyocera International, Inc.
www.kyocerasolar.com

Sierra Solar Systems
www.sierrasolar.com

Backwoods Solar electric systems
www.backwoodssolar.com

Wind Turbines

Ampair
www.ampair.com
This British firm has reliable and durable products. The Pacific 100 Hawk is one of the best units available for emergency battery charging.

Composting Toilets

The time has come to mulch and compost and at the same time prepare for sewer and water supply problems. See Chapters 11 and 24 for further information.

BioLet USA, Inc.
740.498.4073
www.biolet.com

Clivus Multrum Composting Toilets
www.clivusmultrum.com

Sun-Mar Corp
www.sun-mar.com

Envirolet Composting Toilet Systems
www.envirolet.com

Nuk-Alert

KI4U Inc.
830.672-8734
www.ki4u.com
During a nuclear emergency of any type, your survival will depend upon your ability to detect radiation levels. Consider a NukAlert detector as a first line of protection against nuclear terrorism and "dirty bombs." See Chapter 22: Nuclear and Radiological Events.

Storm/Emergency Shelters

With a mind paid to riding out extreme weather conditions of the 21st-century.

Radius Engineering
972.552.2484   fax: 972.552.2485
www.bombshelters.com

Storm and Tornado Shelters of Texas
www.shelters-of-texas.com

Disaster-Resistant Homes

Steel-Reinforced Concrete Domes

Monolithic Domes
972.483.7423
www.monolithic.com
Monolithic Domes of Italy, Texas specializes in the construction of steel-reinforced concrete domes of any size and shape. Highly disaster-resistant, they're completely fireproof and energy efficient.

Formworks Building Co.
970.247.2100
www.formworksbuilding.com
Called "Nest Eggs," these homes are designed to be earth-covered to add to disaster resistance. Strong and energy-efficient, Nest Eggs are said to have a life span of 200 to 1,000 years.

Geodesic Domes (Steel-reinforced Concrete)

American Ingenuity, Inc.
www.aidomes.com
American Ingenuity produces traditional-style Geodesic Dome kits that are inexpensive and easy to build.

Quick and Inexpensive Geodesic Domes

Pacific Domes
888.488.8127 or 541.488.7737
www.pacificdomes.com
Pacific Domes has been in the Geodesic dome-building business for nearly three decades. They're durable, inexpensive, and aesthetically pleasing, designed to blend into nature.

Shelter Systems
650.323.6202.
www.shelter-systems.com
These geodesic structures have their own tarp fasteners called "Grip Clips," and they make great temporary emergency disaster shelters.

Wood Frame Geodomes

Timberline Geodesics
www.domehome.com

Oregon Dome Inc.
www.domes.com

Natural Spaces Domes
www.naturalspacesdomes.com

Alternative Homebuilding Books

The Solar House: Passive Heating and Cooling by Dan Chiras
Home Work: Handbuilt Shelter by Lloyd Kahn
The Complete Book of Underground Houses by Rob Roy
Do Your Own Wiring by K. E. Armpriester
Do-it-Yourself Plumbing by Max Alth
The Home Water Supply by Stu Campbell
The Independent Home by Michael Potts
Wells and Septic Systems by Max Alth
The Home Water Supply by Stu Campbell
Natural Home Heating by Greg Pahl
Clean House, Clean Planet by Karen Logan

Emergency Preparedness and Survival Websites

Mother Earth Magazine
www.motherearthnews.com
There is no better resource to help you assemble all of the information and materials you need to build an independent homestead.

ModernSurvival.net
ModernSurvival.net is considered the bible of modern emergency preparedness practitioners. The online magazine is chock full of information about all aspects of emergency preparedness and survival. You must subscribe for full access.

EquippedToSurvive.com
This site reviews the best outdoor equipment, and posts useful emergency preparedness, search and rescue and survival information.

Survival.com
This site has great "real deal" information about emergency preparedness and outdoor survival.

SurvivalRing.org
The Survival Ring is a group of websites linked together to provide up-to-date and practical information about all aspects of emergency preparedness and survival.

Selected Bibliography

Alibek, Ken, *Biohazard*. Delta Books, 2000.

Alibek, Ken, *et al., Jane's Chem-Bio Handbook*. Jane's Information Group 2nd ed., 2002.

"American Survival Guide," January 2000, February 1998, November 1994.

Anderson, Paul, *Omega: Murder of the Ecosystem and Suicide of Man*. Wm. C. Brown Co., 1971.

Armistead, Leigh, *Information Operations: Warfare and the Hard Reality of Soft Power (Issues in Twenty-First Century Warfare)*. Potomac, 2004.

Arnold, Daniel, *The Great Bust Ahead*. Vorago-U.S., 2002.

Bhaktivedanta Swami Prabhupada, A.C., *A Higher Taste*. Bhaktivedanta Book Trust, 1991.

Bonner, William, & Addison Whiggin. *Financial Reckoning Day: Surviving the Soft Depression of the 21st Century*. John Wiley & Sons, 2003.

Brown, F., *Chemical Warfare: A Study in Restraints*. Princeton University Press, 1968.

Brown, Sarah, *The Best of Vegetarian Cuisine*. Random House, 1985.

Caldicott, Helen., *The Arms Race and Nuclear War*. William Morrow and Co., 1984.

Clarfield, H. Gerard, & Wiecek, William M., *Nuclear America: Military and Civilian Nuclear Power in the United States 1940–1980*. Harper & Row, 1984.

Cockburn, Andrew & Leslie, *One Point Safe*. Little, Brown, 1997.

Colborn, Theo, *et al., Our Stolen Future: How We Are Threatening Our Fertility, Intelligence and Survival*. Plume, 1997.

Cookson, John, & Judith Nottingham, *A Survey of Chemical and Biological Warfare*. Monthly Review Press, 1969, 1970.

Cooper, Kenneth, *Aerobics*. Bantam, 1981.

Cornwell, Kevin D., *Ham Radio Simplified*. Global Oceanic Communication, Education & Assistance Network, 1998.

Department of Defense, *U.S. Army Survival Manual: FM 21-26*. 1970–1990.

Ehrlich, H. Anne, & John W. Birks, *Hidden Dangers: Environmental Consequences of Preparing for War*. Sierra Club Books, 1990.

Fears, J. Wayne, *The Complete Book of Outdoor Survival*. Krause Publications; rev. ed., 2000.

FEMA, *Are You Ready: An In-Depth Guide to Citizen Preparedness*, 2002. [Warning: not as in-depth as the subtitle would have you believe.]

————, *Emergency Preparedness U.S.A.,* 1994.

Forsberg, Krister, and S. D. Mansdoff, *Quick Selection Guide to Chemical Protective Clothing*. Wiley; 4th ed., 2003.

Fuller, Buckminster R., *Design for the Real World: Human Ecology and Social Change*, Pantheon, 1972.

————, *Operations Manual for Spaceship Earth*. Pocket Books, 1971.

————, *Synergetics*. MacMillan, 1982.

————, *Utopia or Oblivion: The Prospects For Humanity*. Bantam Books, 1969.

Garrett, Laurie, *The Coming Plague*. Penguin, 1995.

Gipe, Paul, *Wind Energy Basics: A Guide to Small and Micro Wind Systems*. Chelsea Green Publishing Company, 1999.

Harris, Robert, & Jeremy Paxman, *A Higher Form of Killing: The Secret Story of Chemical and Biological Warfare*. Beech Tree Books, 1988.

Hatfield, Fred, *Power*. McGraw Hill, 1989.

Hersh, S. M., *Chemical and Biological Warfare: America's Hidden Arsenal*. Bobbs-Merrill, 1968.

Joy, Bill, "Why the Future Doesn't Need Us," *Wired* 8.04, April 2000.

Kincaid, Reid, *Extreme Survival Almanac: Everything You Need to Know to Live Through a Shipwreck, Plane Crash, or Any Outdoor Crisis Imaginable*. Paladin Press, 2002.

Kresson, Kearny H., *Nuclear War Survival Skills*. Oregon Institute of Science & Medicine; 4th rep. ed. 1999.

Livingstone, C. Neal, & Joseph D. Douglass, Jr., *CBW: The Poor Man's Atomic Bomb*. Institute for Foreign Policy Analysis, 1984.

Marks, John, *The Search for the Manchurian Candidate: The CIA and Mind Control*. Times Books, 1979.

Marquette, Stephen, & Jeffrey Adams, *First Responder's Guide to Weapons of Mass Destruction (WMD): Practical Techniques and Procedures for Responding to a Terrorist Incident Involving WMD*. American Society for Industrial Security, 2001.

McDermott, Jeanne, *The Killing Winds*. Arbor House, 1987.

National Institutes of Health. *Clinical Guidelines on the Identification, Evaluation, and Treatment of Overweight and Obesity in Adults.* National Heart, Lung, and Blood Institute, 1998.

Nero, Anthony V., *A Guidebook to Nuclear Reactors*. University of California Press, 1979.

NIOSH Pocket Guide to Chemical Hazards. J.J. Keller, 2003

Pillar & Yamamoto, "Army Gives a Boost to Exotic, Non-Lethal Weapons," *Defense Week*, October 19, 1992.

Pillar, Charles, and R. Keith Yamamoto, *Gene Wars: Military Control over the New Genetic Technologies*. Beech Tree Books, 1988.

Preston, Richard, *Crisis in the Hot Zone*. Anchor Books, 1995.

The Problem of Chemical and Biological Warfare: CB Weapons Today. Stockholm International Peace Research Institute, 1973.

Ramsey, Dan, *The Complete Idiot's Guide to Solar Power for Your Home*. Alpha Books, 2002.

Report of the Chemical Warfare Commission. U.S. Government Printing Office, 1985.

Rheingold, Howard, *The Millennium Whole Earth Catalog*. HarperCollins, 1994.

Rose, William, *A Survey of Entomological Warfare*. 1981 U.S. Army Technical Report (unclassified), 1981.

Roy, Rob, *The Complete Book of Underground Houses*. Sterling, 1994.

Ryan, Frank, *Virus X: Tracking the New Killer Plagues*. Back Bay Books, 1998.

Schaffer, John, & Doug Pratt, *Real Goods Solar Living Source Book: The Complete Guide to Renewable Energy Technologies and Sustainable Living*. Gaiam Real Goods; 11th ed., 2001.

Schell, Jonathan. *Fate of the Earth*, Stanford University Press, 2000.

Schuh, Dwight R., *Modern Survival: Outdoor Gear and Savvy to Bring You Back Alive*. D. McKay Co., 1979.

Simkin, Tom, & Lee Siebert, *Volcanoes of the World*. Geoscience Press; 2nd ed., 1995.

Strong, Stephen J., *The Solar Electric House: Energy for the Environmentally-Responsive, Energy-Independent Home*. Sustainability Press, 1994.

Stunkard A.J., and T. A. Wadden, eds., *Obesity: Theory and Therapy*. Raven Press; 2nd ed., 1993.

Suzuki, David, & Anita Gordon, *It's a Matter of Survival*. Stoddart Publishing Co., Toronto, 1990.

Tsipis, Kosta, *Arsenal: Understanding Weapons in the Nuclear Age*. Simon & Shuster, 1983.

Turco, R., & C. Sagan, "Nuclear Winter: Global Consequences of Multiple Nuclear Explosions," *Science* 222, 1983.

Unied States, Senate Select Subcommittee on Health and Scientific Research, *Biological Testing Involving Human Subjects by the Department of Defense*. 1977.

U.S. Department of Energy, Final Environmental Impact Statement, Special Isotope Separation Project, 1988.

U.S. Government, *21st Century Complete Guide to Bioterrorism, Biological and Chemical Weapons, Germs and Germ Warfare, Nuclear and Radiation Terrorism*. Progressive Management, 2001.

Wells, H.G., *The Shape of Things to Come*. 1933.

Weiss, Eric A., *A Comprehensive Guide to Wilderness and Travel Medicine*. Adventure Medical Kits 1992–1997

Woodwell G. M., *The Biotic Effects of Ionizing Radiation*. Ambio, 1982.

Worldwatch, *State of the World*. W. W. Norton & Co., 1988.

Youth International Party Information Service, *Blacklisted News, Secret History: From Chicago '68 to 1984*. 1983.

Zebrowski, Ernest Jr., *Perils of a Restless Planet: Scientific Perspectives on Natural Disasters*. Cambridge U.P., 1997.

Preparedness Checklist

All checklists are available to download and print at **www.PreparednessNow.net**

Home Preparedness Supplies

Water
Three gallons of water per person per day for a three-day supply should be your minimum. A 14-day supply is suggested. For further information about water supplies, their storage and purification, see Chapter 7.

Mark down the amount and location of your water below:
Amount of water: _____
Storage Area: _____

Food
Store a three-week supply that can feed each member of your household with 1800 calories per day. For information about food supplies and their storage, see Chapter 7.

Mark below the foods, quantity and area where you're storing the food.
Foods and Quantity: _____
_____
_____
Storage Area: _____
_____

Medicine
If your medications require refrigeration, invest in a battery-powered refrigerator (see Chapter 12). Types of medication you (or your family) need and where you store them:

Med: _____ **Stored:** _____ **Exp:** _____
Med: _____ **Stored:** _____ **Exp:** _____
Med: _____ **Stored:** _____ **Exp:** _____
Med: _____ **Stored:** _____ **Exp:** _____
Med: _____ **Stored:** _____ **Exp:** _____
Med: _____ **Stored:** _____ **Exp:** _____

Essential Items for the Home

☐ **Grab-and-Go Bag** Storage Area: _____

☐ **E-Kit** (Should be near you at all times)

☐ **Battery-free flashlights** (and extra bulbs) Storage Area: _____

☐ **Battery-free radio(s)** Storage Area: _____

☐ **Cord, rope, twine** Storage Area: _____

☐ **Duct tape** Storage Area: _____

☐ **Emergency stove and fuel** Storage Area: _____

☐ **Emergency transportation** Storage Area:_____

☐ **Fire extinguisher(s)** Storage Area: _____

☐ **First aid kit** Storage Area:_____

☐ **Insect repellent** Storage Area: _____

☐ **Knife (full tang)** Storage Area: _____

☐ **Lantern(s)** (battery, solar, or kerosene) Storage Area: _____

☐ **Matches** Storage Area: _____

☐ **NukAlert or radiation dose rate meter** Storage Area: _____

☐ **N,P,R -100, 95 respirator masks** Storage Area: _____

☐ **Protective clothing** Storage Area: _____

☐ **Pry bar** Storage Area:_____

☐ **Self-defense equipment** Storage Area: _____

☐ **Sewing kit** Storage Area:_____

☐ **Sleeping bags/blankets** Storage Area:_____

☐ **Smoke escape hoods** Storage Area: _____

☐ **Tent(s)** Storage Area:_____

☐ **Tent patch kit** Storage Area: _____

☐ **Tool kit** Storage Area: _____

☐ **Utensils** Storage Area(s): _____

☐ **Water containers** Storage Area(s): _____

☐ **Water filters** Storage Area: _____

☐ **Work gloves** Storage Area: _____

Recommended Items

☐ **Bicycle trailer** Storage Area: _____

☐ **Emergency heater** Storage Area:_____

☐ **Gas masks** Storage Area: _____

☐ **Generator (solar, gas, diesel)** Storage Area: _____

☐ **Hatchet** Storage Area: _____

☐ **PAPR masks** Storage Area:_____

☐ **Radio scanner** Storage Area: _____

❑ **Spare rechargeable batteries** Storage Area: _____

❑ **Solar battery recharger** Storage Area: _____

❑ **Two-way radio transmitters** Storage Area: _____

Personal Hygiene

❑ **Denture cream, Depends undergarments** (for the elderly or ill)

❑ **Moist towelettes or baby wipes**

❑ **Mouthwash, floss**

❑ **Toothbrushes, toothpaste**

❑ **Soap, shampoo, deodorant (Lavelin)**

❑ **Shaving lotion, razors, lotion**

❑ **Small mirror**

❑ **Tampons, sanitary napkins**

If You Have a Baby or Infant Add:

❑ **Baby powder, shampoo, lotion, ointments**

❑ **Bottles with extra nipples**

❑ **Baby pillow, blankets, sheets**

❑ **Baby toys**

❑ **Colic remedies (Pediacalm, Gripe water)**

❑ **Diapers**

❑ **Extra baby clothes**

❑ **Formula, milk (powdered, soy, rice)**

❑ **Rubber pads**

❑ **Small portable crib**

❑ **Teething ring**

Personal Emergency Supplies

❑ **Extra pair of prescription glasses and/or contact lenses with solution**

❑ **Emergency clothing:**

❑ **Boots**

❑ **5 pairs of underwear**

❑ **Socks**

❑ **3 shirts**

❑ **2 pairs of loose-fitting pants**

❑ **Raingear**

❑ **Hat** (baseball caps, boonie hats, etc.)

☐ **Fisherman's or tactical vest** (to store extra preparedness items)
☐ **Playing cards, CD players (with CDs), iPod, mini-video games with extra batteries**

Sanitation

☐ **Bucket** (five gallon) with lid
☐ **Cat litter** (odor-removing) for solid human waste
☐ **Disinfectants** (Lysol, Encore, Clorox)
☐ **Garbage bags** (heavy-duty) for lining the bucket
☐ **Shovel** (small size, or scoop)
☐ **Soap, detergent** (preferably in liquid form)
☐ **Toilet paper**
☐ **Toilet seat** for top of bucket

Special Optional Preparedness Gear

☐ **Fire escape ladder** (for home or office) Storage Area _____
☐ **Gas chainsaw** (for fallen trees, utility poles) Storage Area_____
☐ **Inflatable raft** (for frequent floods) Storage Area_____
☐ **Pulley system and rope** (for heavy lifting) Storage Area _____

Basic E-Kit
See Chapter 3, page 36 for item descriptions.

Essential Items

☐ **E-Kit pouch**
☐ **EMT tool pouch**
☐ **Flashlight**
☐ **Multi-tool**
☐ **Mini-pry bar or 4-way hatchet tool**
☐ **Small first aid pouch kit**
☐ **Smoke mask**
☐ **Whistle**

Recommended Items

- ❏ **Butane lighter**
- ❏ **Cord**
- ❏ **EMT shears**
- ❏ **One box weatherproof matches**

Grab-and-Go Bag for Home

See Chapter 4, p. 67 for item descriptions.

Essential Items

- ❏ **Backpack/gear bag**
- ❏ **Water containers,** (canteens, camelback jugs) and at least two liters of water per person
- ❏ **Portable water filter, purifier, or water purification tablets**
- ❏ **Emergency food.** Select for nutrition, weight, ease of preparation
- ❏ **Stainless steel mess kit** or outdoor cooking gear
- ❏ **Utensils:** cups, forks, knives, plastic plates
- ❏ **Prescription medication, eyeglasses,** and other special needs items, like contact lens solutions, and hearing aid batteries
- ❏ **Items for infants,** such as formula, diapers, bottles, and pacifiers
- ❏ **Extra set of keys** to your home and car
- ❏ **Documents:** duplicates of all your most important records
- ❏ **Birth, marriage and death certificates**
- ❏ **Driver's license, Social Security card**
- ❏ **Savings and checking account info**
- ❏ **Wills, deeds**
- ❏ **Insurance information**
- ❏ **Mortgages, stocks, bonds, investments info**
- ❏ **Precious photos and jewelry**
- ❏ **Money**
- ❏ **First aid kit**
- ❏ **Tent**
- ❏ **Tarp**
- ❏ **Lighter(s)**
- ❏ **Two Nuwick 120-hour emergency candles**
- ❏ **Weatherproof matches with case**
- ❏ **Two flashlights:** one large, one small, with the large one strapped to the outside of your bag for easy access. Non-incendive are best

- ❏ **Emergency radio:** hand crank or solar only
- ❏ **Crowbar or four-way hatchet tool**
- ❏ **Roll of duct tape**
- ❏ **550-lb. test nylon cord**
- ❏ **Insect repellent**
- ❏ **Clothing detergent:** a small bottle of concentrated liquid such as Tide
- ❏ **Essential toiletries:** soap, shampoo, toothbrush and toothpaste, sunscreen, skin lotion, foot powder, deodorant, feminine hygiene items (for women), baby wipes or toilet paper
- ❏ **Sleeping mat:** inflatable or regular
- ❏ **Heavy-duty plastic garbage bags** for waste disposal
- ❏ **Ziploc storage bags** for waste disposal
- ❏ **Small can of Lysol** or other industrial strength disinfectant for sanitation purposes
- ❏ **Rain ponchos** (lashed to the outside of your bag)
- ❏ **Hats** for each family member
- ❏ **Goggles, military style** (for emergency eye protection)
- ❏ **Sewing kit**
- ❏ **Knife** (full tang)
- ❏ **Sharpening tool**

Recommended Items:

- ❏ **Tube of seam grip** (for emergency tent repair)
- ❏ **Work gloves**
- ❏ **Tri-fold shovel**
- ❏ **Section of stainless steel bailing wire** (used for repairs, e.g. of broken glasses)
- ❏ **Six to 10 ALICE clips**
- ❏ **Two signal mirrors**
- ❏ **Pistol belt**
- ❏ **Combat suspender**
- ❏ **Portable stove** (multi-fuel is best)
- ❏ **Stove fuel and fuel bottles**
- ❏ **Pack of fish hooks**
- ❏ **Five assorted sinkers**
- ❏ **Spool of 30-lb. test fishing line**
- ❏ **Candle lantern**
- ❏ **Cat litter** (for sanitation purposes, to be carried on your hand cart)
- ❏ **Chlorophyll to reduce smell of waster material**
- ❏ **Extra cotton underwear**

- ❏ **Three pairs of wick-dry socks**
- ❏ **Two pairs of seal socks**
- ❏ **Two pairs of Sorbothane shock soles**
- ❏ **Extra pair of sturdy shoes** (tied to the outside of the backpack)
- ❏ **Two pairs of comfortable work pants**
- ❏ **Non-essential toiletries:** foot powder, shampoo, razors and small can of shaving lotion
- ❏ **Sunglasses**
- ❏ **Powdered drink mix, tea, coffee, etc**
- ❏ **Mini-folding chair**
- ❏ **Magnesium fire starter**
- ❏ **Safety or construction helmet** for seismic emergencies

Grab-and-Go Bag for the Office

Essential Items

- ❏ **Bottle(s) of water**
- ❏ **Energy bars**
- ❏ **Flashlight** (non-incendive)
- ❏ **Small emergency radio**
- ❏ **Mini-pry bar** (if you don't include it in your E-Kit)
- ❏ **Small first aid kit**
- ❏ **Emergency rain poncho**
- ❏ **Smoke hood** (even if you have one in your main E-Kit)
- ❏ **Small roll of duct tape**
- ❏ **550-lb. test cord**
- ❏ **Extra keys** (to your home and vehicle)
- ❏ **Extra medication** (if needed)
- ❏ **Extra ID**
- ❏ **Money**

Recommended Items

- ❏ **Change of Clothes (if possible)**
- ❏ **Extra Glasses (if needed)**

Grab-and-Go Bag for Your Car

Essential Items

- ❏ **Sturdy backpack** to store away all your gear
- ❏ **Water** (five gallons at least)
- ❏ **Non-perishable food**
- ❏ **First aid kit** (full size with CPR kit)
- ❏ **Flashlight**
- ❏ **Blankets**
- ❏ **Road flares**
- ❏ **Spare tire and jack, and non-explosive emergency flat fixer**
- ❏ **Road maps of your area and surrounding areas**
- ❏ **Kitty litter, small trash bags, baby wipes, empty water container with a sealable cap and bedpan**
- ❏ **Extra pair of comfortable shoes and change of clothes**
- ❏ **Self-defense equipment** (pepper spray, mace, stun or taser weapon)
- ❏ **Towing line or chain**
- ❏ **Small fire** extinguisher mounted inside the passenger compartment
- ❏ **Soap and other toiletries**
- ❏ **Emergency battery charger**
- ❏ **550-lb. test cord**
- ❏ **Money**

Recommended items

- ❏ **Photovoltaic trickle battery charger**
- ❏ **Radio scanner** (see emergency communications section)
- ❏ **Tri-folding shovel**
- ❏ **Reading material, playing cards, CDs**
- ❏ **Car air freshener**
- ❏ **Sunglasses**
- ❏ **See items from Home Grab-and-Go Bag**

Emergency Evacuation Cards are available to download and print at
www.PreparednessNow.net

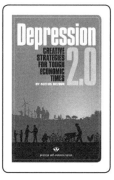
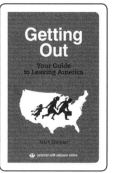
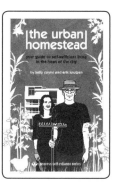

Notes

....
....
....
....
....
....
....
....
....

Notes

Notes

Notes

Notes

Notes

Notes

Notes